CULTURAL PATTERNS AND NEUROCOGNITIVE CIRCUITS

East–West Connections

Exploring Complexity

For four centuries our sciences have progressed by looking at its objects of study in a reductionist manner. In contrast complexity science, that has been evolving during the last 30–40 years, seeks to look at its objects of study from the bottom up, seeing them as systems of interacting elements that form, change, and evolve over time. Complexity therefore is not so much a subject of research as a way of looking at systems. It is inherently interdisciplinary, meaning that it gets its problems from the real non-disciplinary world and its energy and ideas from all fields of science, at the same time affecting each of these fields.

The purpose of this series on complexity science is to provide insights in the development of the science and its applications, the contexts within which it evolved and evolves, the main players in the field and the influence it has on other sciences.

Volume 1: Aha.... That is Interesting!
John Holland, 85 Years Young
edited by Jan W Vasbinder

Volume 2: Cultural Patterns and Neurocognitive Circuits:
East–West Connections
edited by Jan W Vasbinder & Balázs Gulyás

CULTURAL PATTERNS AND NEUROCOGNITIVE CIRCUITS

East–West Connections

Editors

Jan W. Vasbinder
Balázs Gulyás
NTU, Singapore

World Scientific

NEW JERSEY • LONDON • SINGAPORE • BEIJING • SHANGHAI • HONG KONG • TAIPEI • CHENNAI • TOKYO

Published by

World Scientific Publishing Co. Pte. Ltd.
5 Toh Tuck Link, Singapore 596224
USA office: 27 Warren Street, Suite 401-402, Hackensack, NJ 07601
UK office: 57 Shelton Street, Covent Garden, London WC2H 9HE

British Library Cataloguing-in-Publication Data
A catalogue record for this book is available from the British Library.

Exploring Complexity — Volume 2
CULTURAL PATTERNS AND NEUROCOGNITIVE CIRCUITS
East–West Connections

ISBN 978-981-3147-48-5

Printed in Singapore

Contents

Introduction

Jan Vasbinder and Balázs Gulyás

Oh, East is East, and West is West, and never the twain shall meet,
Till Earth and Sky stand presently at God's great Judgment Seat;
But there is neither East nor West, Border, nor Breed, nor Birth,
When two strong men stand face to face, though they come from the ends of the earth!

The Ballad of East and West
Rudyard Kipling (1889)

East and West, two major worlds of aspirations, cultures, world-views, theoretical and practical approaches to life and death, are in the focus of the exploratory activities of Para Limes, which already started a systematic exploration of the similarities and differences between the cultural-cognitive-behavioural-emotional patterns of the East and the West, with special regard to their neurobiological underpinnings in the human brain.

A question, which is raised often by each and every individual on Earth, namely "What, in the thoughts and heart of an individual person, makes his/her life worth living?" is also coming into the fore among the topics to be explored by the Para Limes Institute, as this question is often asked but rarely answered in a meticulous scientific manner. In this spirit, the present workshop would explore various aspects of "a good life", including cultural, neurocognitive, emotional aspects as well as the Eastern and Western approaches, and it will focus on cultural patterns and cognitive patterns in the East and West, with special regard to those patterns which are determined by our natural-genetic endowments in contrast to those patterns which are influenced by our cultural ("East-West") influences. Within this context, a unique flavour will be given during the talks and discussion to "a good life", "a life worth living" aspects.

In line with the aspirations of Para Limes, with the present workshop we intend to continue our interdisciplinary and intercultural approach in which boundaries of disciplines and institutes should not limit the scope of the individual talks or the discussions. Hence we have invited speakers from fundamentally different fields to make sure we have mind boggling - mind broadening discussions.

Common sense is the most fairly distributed thing in the world, for each one thinks he is so well-endowed with it that even those who are hardest to satisfy in all other matters are not in the habit of desiring more of it than they already have.

The Para Limes Institute at Nanyang Technological University is dedicated to exploring complexity by going beyond the boundaries of disciplines, cultures and institutions. In this spirit, Para Limes has initiated exploratory projects by teams of world-class scientists, philosophers, artists, policy makers, and men and women of practice and it has already organised a series of conferences on various interdisciplinary themes, related to its mission.

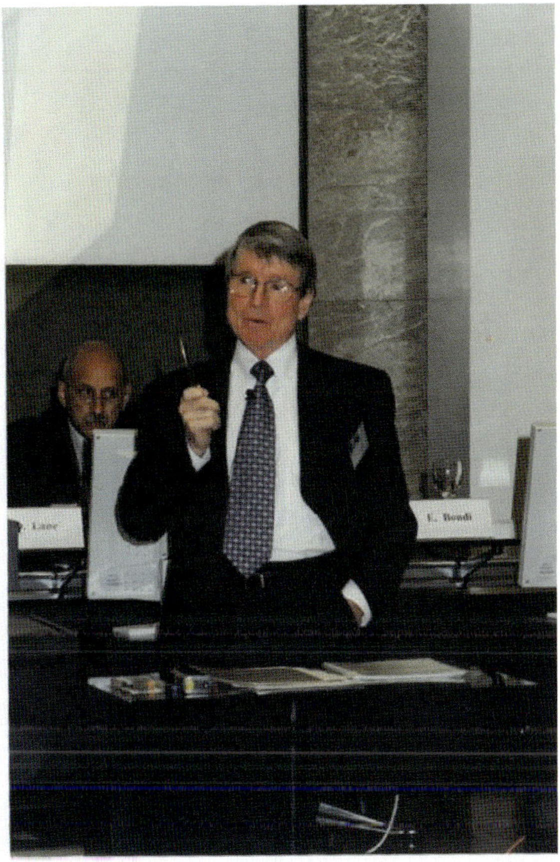

Prof John H. Holland died on August 9, 2015. He was an explorer and a pioneer who established complexity research as a new field of science. He was blessed with an inexhaustible flow of original ideas. His work and views on complex adaptive systems, computation, evolution and cognition have influenced a broad field of sciences, as varied as psychology, neuroscience, economics and linguistics.

The lecture "*Cycles and Hierarchies"* he gave at the conference *"East West connections, cultural circuits in the brain*" was his last public lecture. He did not have time anymore to write up the paper for this book.

To honor him we have transcribed the videotape we made of his lecture and included the text, together with the figures he presented during his lecture, in this volume.

1 Cycles and Hierarchies

John H. Holland (1929-2015)

Balázs Gulyás (BG): Let me introduce to you now our distinguished guest and discussion partner, Professor John Holland. And let me start my introduction with a reference to one slide which we saw yesterday in Per Roland's lecture. Per showed a black and white snapshot of an eminent nineteenth century German scientist, the polymath genius Hermann von Helmholtz, who — according to Per — looked very tired because he had just finished a very long book... I am happy to inform you that Hermann von Helmholtz's great-great-great-great-grandson is here with us today.

Do you know all this, John? I have checked on the Mathematics Genealogy Project website who your ancestors are and I had to realize that your great-great-great-great-grandfather was the named Hermann von Helmholtz whose student was Wilhelm Wundt, the leading psychologist of his age and the father of experimental psychology, and you're the great-great-great-grandson of Wundt. (https://www.genealogy.math.ndsu.nodak.edu/id.php?id=5064).

John H. Holland (JHH): Indeed, we know there are only six steps between any person...

Let me start my lecture by this very standard diagram, so that we have at least a similar terminology. We have got the body of the neuron, we got the axon and one thing to really keep in mind is every single neuron touches about 10,000 other neurons (Fig. 1).

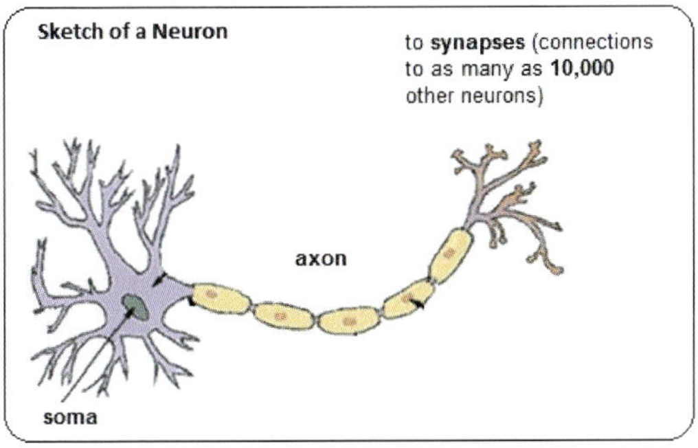

Fig. 1.

The thing that I want to talk about is the number of loops in the central nervous system. If we look at the neocortex, we see that we have approximately 500,000 columns with 70,000 neurons in the columns. A piece of cortex, the size of grain salt, contains 680 fibers and 774 synapses. Because there are 1,000 more synapses per neuron, and this is the key point, all possible loops, defined by selecting neurons two-at-a-time, three-at-a-time, up to length 25. So all possible paths, all possible loops of length 25 or so, will be present there (Fig. 2).

Organization of the Neocortex

Neurons in the human neocortex are organized in

500,000 columns (0.5mm diameter/2mm depth)
~70,000 neurons in each column.

The columns are divided into six layers, I through VI:

Layers I-III provide cross and intra-column connections.
Layer IV primarily receives incoming sensory information.
Layers V-VI primarily project out of cortex.

Recent details: *Science* 342 (22 Nov. 2013) (Jeff Lichtman – Harvard)
"(A) salt grain-sized ... cylinder of (mouse tissue contains) 680 nerve fivers ... and 774 synapses ..."

Fig. 2.

The point is that if I start talking about consciousness, about the kind of things that we expect of a human - to look ahead, look at alternatives, to try out alternatives, to keep things in mind - all that depends on the number of loops. And all these loops, up to about 25 lengths, are present in the neocortex (Fig. 3).

The Prevalence of Loops in Neocortex (2)

Because there are 1,000 or more synapses per neuron,
all possible loops, defined by selecting neurons 2-at-a-time, 3-at-a-time, up to length 25 or so, will be present in a grain of salt-sized region.

A calculation using the binomial theorem shows that there are over
10 billion distinct directed loops in this salt-sized region.

Fig. 3.

The neurons have a time-varying threshold which is not fixed. The longer it is between times that a neuron fires, the easier it is to fire it. So the neurons are sitting there, waiting to be fired, and if you ignore them for a long time, then eventually they will fire on their own. If they have been firing at higher rate, they develop a fatigue and they are more and more difficult to fire. This means that in the long run the neurons tend to fire at some average rate. Sometimes fast, sometimes slow.

A key point in this context is the rule established by Donald Hebb which says that if A fires and B immediately fires afterward, then the synaptic connection between them gets stronger. If A fires and B does not fire, then the connection gets weaker. The more, they can become inhibitory to prevent the following neuron from firing (Fig. 4).

Properties of Neuron Relevant to Recirculation of Spikes in Loops

Time-varying threshold

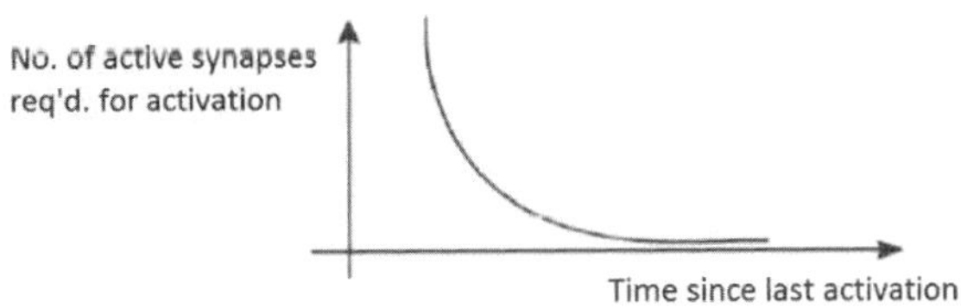

Fatigue (increasing threshold based on firing rate)

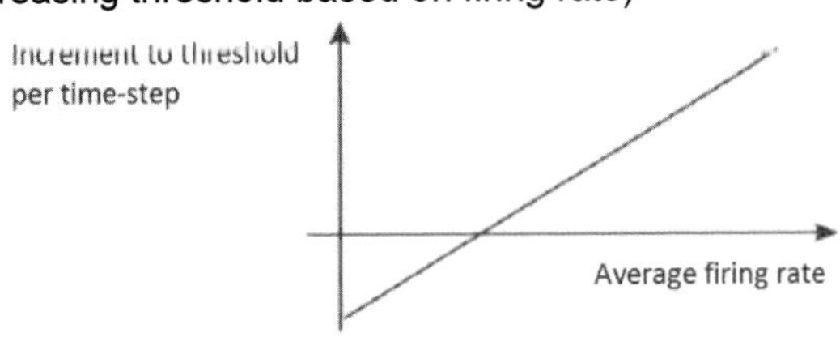

Hebb's learning rule

When neuron A is directly connected to neuron B

If A fires and **B fires immediately** afterward (~1msec):

then the **connection between A and B is strengthened.**

If A fires and **B does not fire immediately** afterward

then the **connection between A and B is weakened.**

Fig. 4.

The neurons in self-stimulating loops continue firing until the threshold gets to the point that they are very difficult to fire. A long loop accumulates fatigue more slowly because the neurons are activated more slowly. In subsets of neurons, as shown in Fig. 5, each neuron in the subset fires simultaneously.

The Origin of Loops

A connected set of 3 neurons in a small section of neocortex will make over 1 trillion synaptic contacts. **Many of these contacts will be with the originating 3 neurons, producing loops.**

Loops allow neural pulses to ***recirculate***, so that a given neuron can ***restimulate*** itself via the intervening neurons in the path.

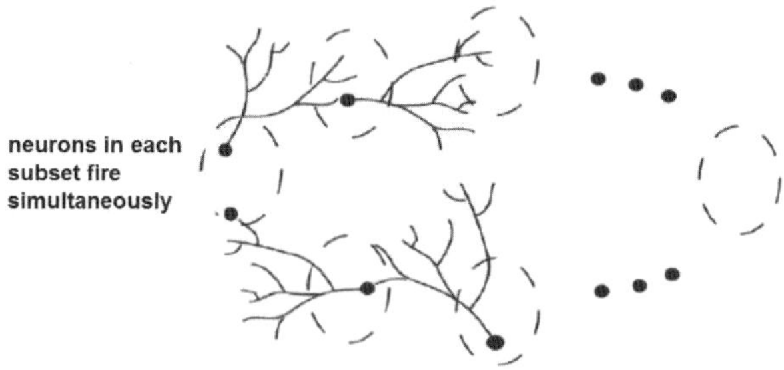

By looking at connected neurons in a small neo-cortical section 2-at-a-time, 3-at-a-time, and so on, it is clear that the section contains a vast number of loops. A calculation using the binomial theorem shows that **there are more than 10^9 distinct loops in a grain-of-salt sized section.**

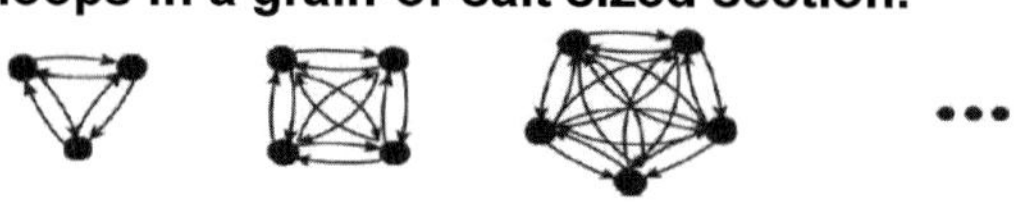

Fig. 5.

This has a lot to do with the way we develop language. I can think of something where I have ‘fetch’ and ‘ball’. The longer loops allow me to express those two things together so that I can now say “fetch ball” or “fetch”-“ball”. And if I then look at this notion of simultaneous spikes to fire a neuron, it will take 20 of those on time-step 3, but 8 of those in time-step 6, simply because of the elapsed time since the neuron last fired (Fig. 6).

A very simple saccade hierarchy (1).

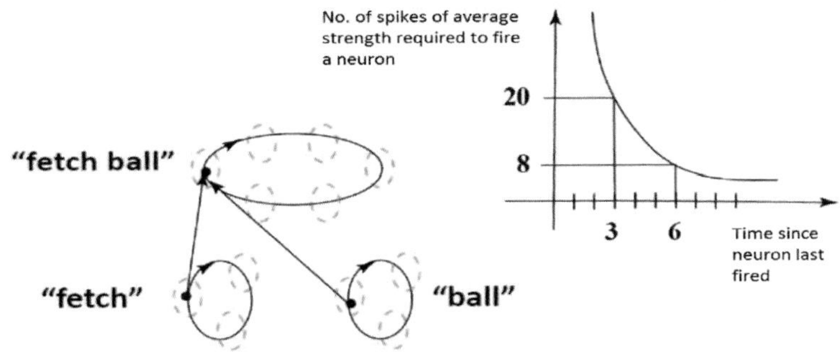

For this example assume all synapses have close to the same strength.

Assume also that:

(i) it takes **20 simultaneous spikes to fire a neuron on time-step 3** (the first time-step after the absolute refractory period).

(ii) it takes **8 simultaneous spikes to fire a neuron on time-step 6** (4 time-steps after the absolute refractory period).

Fig. 6.

The point that I consider very important: These systems at the higher level use these various activities as building blocks to build more complex activities. So this is just like a children's set of building blocks. You have some blocks around and you use them to develop more complex things by simply putting them together (Fig. 7).

Building Blocks

Loop interaction allows various activities (such as utterances) **to act as building blocks for higher order activities** (such as utterance sequences).

Fig. 7.

We should notice the combinatorics of the building blocks and ask ourselves if we have ever watched a child. How does a child build something really complex? Notice that a castle which any child will soon be able to build is one of 1.000,000,000,000 possibilities. How do they get there?

It is really not going to get there at random. And if I look at this, I see that on the other hand, if I have the simple structure of two columns with an archway, that's one out of 4,000. That is something that I can get by random trial and error. So, if we look at the combinatorics of building blocks, what we have to understand is the following: how do we get these very complex structures. The claim is that we get these complex structures by putting together structures that are easier to achieve (Fig. 8).

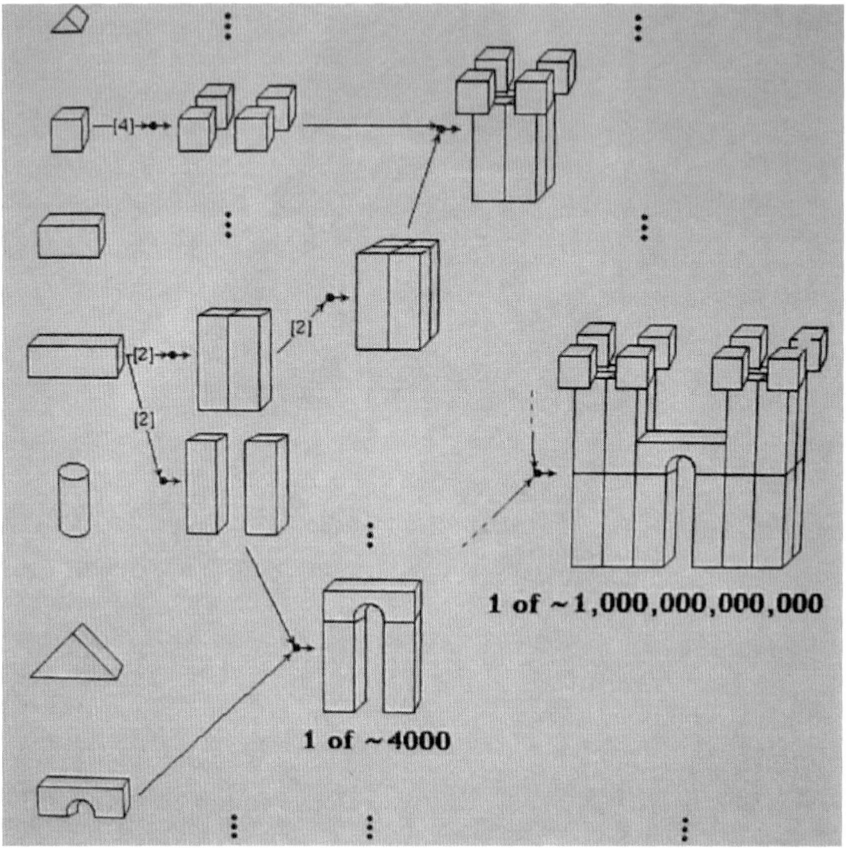

Fig. 8.

Regarding the neocortex: because of the way the system is designed, because there are so many loops in even a small section of the cortex, loops with the desired hierarchical properties of up to 25 lengths will almost always be present.

It is worthwhile noticing here that there are three very different kinds of models and these are rarely distinguished in the literature. (1) There are Data-driven Models and weather prediction is a good example of them. We collect a lot of data and then we try to find correlations and make predictions and so on with that kind of model. (2) Very different kinds of models are the Existence-proof Models. These models are often called Johnny after John von Neumann who used it quite cleverly to show that something is possible. John von Neumann was the first one to show that a machine could reproduce itself. Before that, if you looked at any biology text they said that self-reproduction was a property that distinguishes living organisms from non-living ones. Consequently, textbooks had to be rewritten after Neumann's demonstration of self-reproducing machines. (3) Finally, there are Exploratory Models which try to say something about what might be possible (Fig. 9).

3 Kinds of Models

Data-driven Models
(e.g. weather prediction)

Existence-proof Models
(e.g. von Neumann's self-reproducing machine)

Exploratory Models
(e.g. combinations of well-known mechanisms to form the internal combustion engine)

Fig. 9.

Now, let me talk just a little bit more about the Exploratory Models. If I am looking at this carefully, I have a set of things — I call them gauges from making observations. And if I look at this particular example, there are three gauges each of which has 5 readings. If that is the case, it is possible that the model has 125 states that I have to observe. You can think of these things like, for instance, the control panels on an airplane (Fig. 10).

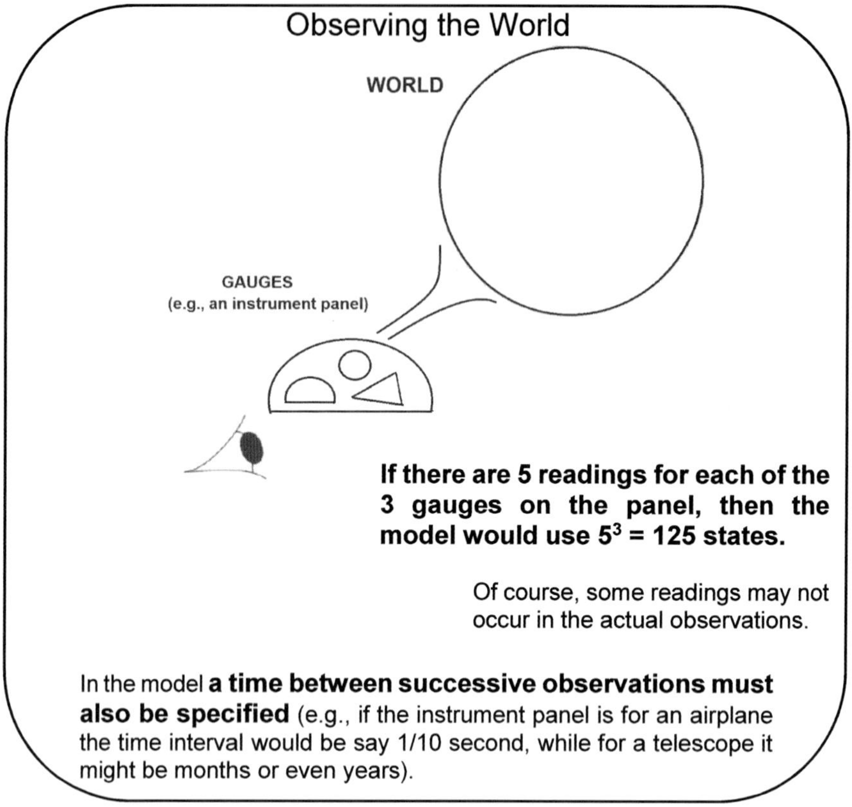

Fig. 10.

Within this context it is ignored sometime that we have to state how long and how frequent are our observations. How much time elapses between one observation and another? Like in a pilot's control panel, each party provides us with an observation every second or so, or it does it even more frequently. On the other hand, if I am observing something like the planets, this process may take years or centuries or in the case of the voyager's spacecraft even longer.

In this sense if a model is valid, then using a set of correct observations, a set of readings, and then the set of changes that my model uses to predict how the world is moving forward, then the model should be the same as the world. Consequently, if I make an observation later in the world, I should get to the same place in the diagram of model. This is what is called communitivity of the diagram. And this is or should be behind every careful notion of what constitutes a valid model: the communitivity of the diagram (Fig. 11).

Models: Reduction and Emergence

The contemplation in natural science of a wider domain than the actual leads to a far better understanding of the actual.

-- A. S. Eddington

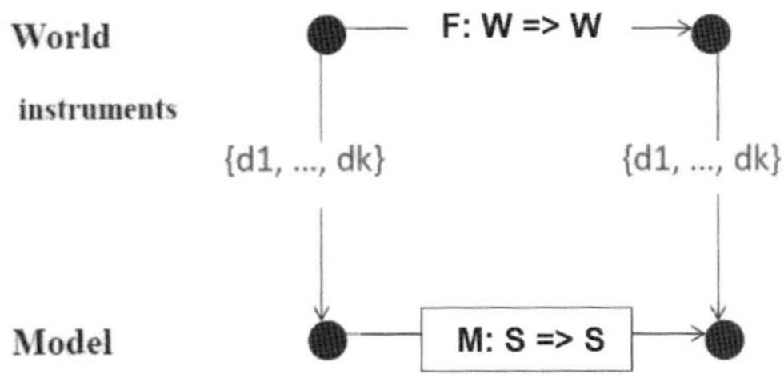

Gell-Mann points out that **3 orders of magnitude** in the scale of observations (e.g. from molecules to fluid flow) requires **new laws**. New laws are ***constrained*** by, but ***not determined*** by, the laws at lower levels.

Fig. 11.

Now, if we use notions to look at the development of language, we see that there is no explicit value assigned to language. This has a lot of consequences. One of the people that I worked with for a long time, Helena Hong Gao, did study this. She is fluent in Chinese, Swedish and English. She has studied young children in each of these language groups and one of the main things she discovered was that in each of these groups the children did not acquire an action word, and this is without exception, until they could do the action. And this says a lot. We know that gesture is important in language. Nobody talks without using their hands, at least nobody that I know. And Helena Hong Gao has obtained experimental data showing it in the aforementioned three groups (Fig. 12).

Objective: An agent-based model of language acquisition and evolution

Each agent's survival depends upon its ability to collect resources that are distributed spatially in its environment.

Language has value to the agent only if it increases the agent's ability to collect these resources.

There's no explicit a priori value assigned to language.

Control experiments are possible: The model can be run with and without language acquisition.

Fig. 12.

Finally, I want to talk briefly about levels of consciousness. At Level 0, we have the things that are 'wired-in', the things that we get just by being human. Regarding this level, the interesting thing is that at this level we have things that are wired-in the brain, and this is true for many animals, too. For instance, if there is a moving object, it attracts our attention. And two people are exposed to the same visual stimulus, we both know that we are looking at the same object. And this is the same, for instance, in a pack of wolves: even if they act as individuals in a pack when seeing a prey, they know that they are looking at the same object. This is a major element of their planning whenever they are trying to single out something to kill. This is built in, wired in their brains (Fig. 13).

Levels of Consciousness – Level 0

'Wired-in' (inherited) cognitive abilities.

Ability to **imitate** utterances and gestures.
Ability to distinguish between **objects** and **actions**.
Awareness of a mutually apprehended **salient** object or action.
Basic **learning** procedures (akin to Hebb's learning rule).

IF (**any signal**) THEN (**random effector activity**)

Fig. 13.

Similarly, just watch your young child: when she moves her hand in front of her face for the first time, she has a big smile. The first time that a baby can control, she reacts with a smile. Based on all these observations you can develop some conditional rules about these wired-in or inherited cognitive abilities. And then you can develop these conditional rules that, for instance, if there is motion in your visual field to the right, move your hand to the right (Fig. 14).

Levels of Consciousness – Level 1

Control of motion (as precursor to gesture).

Task:	Bring hand in controlled motion across visual field.
Mode:	Innate reinforcement for predictable outcomes.
Anticipation:	Movement according to command.

IF (**hand in vision cone**) THEN (**<move hand right>**)

Fig. 14.

We can go level by level of consciousness doing these kinds of things and ultimately, we get to these very language-like actions (Figs. 15, 16, 17).

Levels of Consciousness – Level 2

Utterance for immediate, "wired-in" reward*, e.g. 'Teacher's' smile.*

Task: Social interaction.
Mode: Imitation of situated utterance.
Anticipation: Positive interaction.

IF (**milk bottle present**) THEN (<**utterance "milk"**>)

This rule will be strengtheded, over other random utterances, because **[T-smile] increments sociality reservoir**.

Fig. 15.

Levels of Consciousness – Level 3

Utterance to "move" visible object.

Task: Food acquisition (when food visible).
Mode: Conditioning.
Anticipation: Food.

IF (**milk bottle visible**) THEN (<**"milk"**>)
'Teacher' moves milk bottle to mouth.
IF (<**milk bottle at mouth**>) THEN (<**consume milk**>)

Fig. 16.

Levels of Consciousness – Level 4

Utterance to cause appearance of object.

Task: Food acquisition (when food not visible).
Mode: Internal model (lookahead) – autonomy required.
Anticipation: Appearance of food (later generalized to arbitary objects).

IF ([**hungry**] & **no food visible**) THEN (<**“milk”**>)
'Teacher' acts to fetch milk bottle.
IF (<**T acts** >) THEN (<**milk bottle visible**>)

Acquired from previous levels:
IF (**milk bottle visible**) THEN (<**“milk”**>)
'Teacher' moves milk bottle to mouth.
IF (<**milk bottle at mouth**>) THEN (<**consume milk**>)

Fig. 17.

If we acquire a grammar, the combinatorics starts working for us and these pieces become building blocks that we can put together and get a lot of expressions from a very small vocabulary. For instance, if we have 10 utterances in each of these categories, there are 1,000 meaningful triples and so on (Fig. 18).

Grammars

A grammar makes possible the combinatoric use of vocabulary.

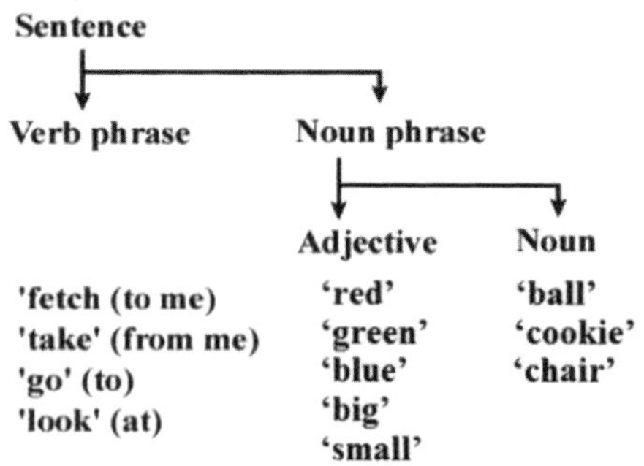

60 meaningful triples can be constructed from the 12 utterances shown.

If there are **10 utterances in each category, 1000 meaningful triples** can be constructed, and so on.

Fig. 18.

And at this point I have to recall what I have already mentioned showed about saccade hierarchy, as I tend to compare the explained grammatic mechanisms with saccades (cfr. Fig. 6), a fundamental mechanism in vision. Our vision does not stare at an object, it always jumps from object to object and this jumping is called saccade. Using similar mechanisms, we can build up a language model (Fig. 19).

Steps in Learning a Proto-Grammar

1) Acquisition of **vocabulary**.

   Babbling (random action) **samples possibilities** (diversity) for attaching utterance to situation.

   Some input invoke **imitation** (e.g., 'shared salient object or action', 'Teacher' utterance)

   'Meaning' emerges from generalization of conditions associated with the same utterance.

2) Acquisition of specific **utterance pairs**.

   Sequences **reduce ambiguity**.

3) **Generalization of sequences** to 'grammatical' rules.

Fig. 19.

Finally, in the next figure I try to highlight the things that we have been doing in order to try to understand the acquisition of language (Fig. 20).

Highlights of Language Model

- The proposed exploratory model is a **signal-processing, agent-based model situated in a environment**.
- The **survival** of the agents, and hence of any **structured proto-linguistic** means of communication, depends upon the agents' **ability to collect resources** in the environment.
- The capacities of any agent are completely determined by a set of **condition/signal rules**.
- Each agent
  - uses general-purpose **triggering mechanisms** (akin to imprinting) to build **default hierarchies**
  - supports goals and sequential action through the formation of **bridging rules**
  - uses a genetic algorithm to explore the space of possible rules by **recombining parts of extant rules**

Fig. 20.

What I propose here is an agent based model. Agents build default hierarchies where you have one very general rule and which is at the top level of the hierarchy. Then you get rules that are exceptions to the general rules, which are acquired and can override the general rule. In other words, the exceptions override the default. And if one looks at this from a point of view of learning, it is relatively easy to develop default hierarchies. The agents use general purpose triggering mechanisms to build these default hierarchies, while support goals and sequential actions through the formation of bridging rules. To create new rules, to make bridging rules are very important actions as this will lead the agent, by using a genetic algorithm, to explore the space of possible rules and by recombining parts of extant rules, to create building blocks and rules again.

BG: Thank you, John.

Do I understand correctly that what you have explained about the emergence of consciousness is a form of emergentism, that is to say, you cannot describe the laws of the new, emergent level by knowing the laws of the lower levels? May I start questioning you regarding Murray Gell-Mann's approach to the so-called "three orders of magnitude change on the observers' point"? Is it, in your opinion, the basis of emergence properties?

JHH: Yeah, I think it is in many cases what is behind the emergence. Gell-Mann's idea is – and you can check it out over and over again – that any time you go through your magnitudes, you get a new set of laws to describe the phenomenon. And to me, that is emergence. For instance, it does it make sense to call an individual molecule wet or not. But if I go up 3 orders of magnitude and get a new set of laws that apply at this new level, for instance in this case the laws for fluid flow laws like the Navier-Stokes equations, I can talk about viscosity. But I am required that the new laws do not violate the constraints imposed by laws at the lower level, 3 orders of magnitude down.

BG: But is it not just a kind of a change in your perspective, your observation point? You go further away of an object or come closer to it and you see some new rules, new characteristics of the same object. If so, the laws depend on the perspective of the observer and not on Nature.

JHH: I think the main point is that if I go from an individual molecule, it makes absolutely no sense that I call it dry or wet, but now I go these 3 orders of magnitude "up", then I get a new set of laws. But they are not violating the constraints imposed by the lower level.

BG: In this context let me raise an issue in which we discussed yesterday: backward causation or downward causation. This is a very controversial idea, but it has been in the field for at least a century or more and there is still quite some misunderstanding and controversy here. The idea is that if you go from a lower level to a higher level, the new rules, the new laws or sets of rules of the higher level do not violate, should not violate those of the lower level. But, and this is the core question behind the idea of backward causation, can the emergent levels have causative influence on the basic constituents at the lower levels?

JHH: Finally, here we get to what I consider the most important activity that I am involved with and these are what I called agent-based models. A simple example of an agent-based model is the stock market. Now, I look at the stock market: the activities of the agents in the market, the people who are buying and selling determine for us the Dow Jones average. But the Dow Jones average also influences what the individual agents do. So it is both top-down and bottom-up in agent-based models and they change over time. I may have an agent there that decides when the market is going up, and I am going to buy or, if the market is dropping, I am going to sell. So agent-based models are the top-down – bottom-up things that can change over time. And we call these adaptive systems complex adaptive systems. And one thing which we know by experiment is that every agent-based model that we look at carefully has, what we call, lever points that with a small amount of action will get big effects. An easy example of that is the vaccine. If I vaccinate, say, for measles, that simple action can have a lifetime effect. So it is a simple lever with big effects. We have as yet absolutely no theory that tells us how to learn about these things.

BG: This appears to be very similar to a philosophical question which has been in forefront of philosophical discussions for many decades. Namely, how can a simple symbol, like a stop signal, initiate a physical reaction, a whole chain of events in the physical world, the stopping of a car or a whole train. And despite the fact that the sign, let it be pictorial or vocal or else, has a very simple information content, it can cause a huge physical event. Is there any theory in general, or do you have any theory about how a symbol can have a 'downward causation effect' or 'backward causation effect' on the physical world?

JHH: This is a question of which we just have no real theory at this point and it is a part of what we need to know a lot more about.

Per Roland: You mentioned the combinatorial possibilities of the child building a castle from the building blocks. There is a very low probability that without any guidance, just by combining the elements randomly, the child can reach the goal. Can one reverse this question with respect to our perception of the surroundings? What I am interested in is the following: Our visual system should be able to identify any object possible, any scenery possible in the surrounding world. Of course, the probability of the possible scenes will vary according to where the observer is. The number of different scenes is a very big number, albeit finite. Yet the visual system is able to see such different scenes.

JHH: I am not sure I would agree with you. I think what I can observe depends on what my instrument panel is. What is it that I am using to make those observations. And that will determine what I can see or not see. If I had the wrong instrument panel, I would not be able to distinguish in the world around us.

Roger Vergauwen: From the way you were talking about language, I have to conclude that language was constructed bottom up, consequently, language is compositional. However, there are theories of language that are non-compositional and there are people who say that some natural languages are not compositional either.

Now my question is very simple. Do you think when you have a choice between the two, that is to say the game-theoretical, non-compositional theories of language and your idea, which would be more correct though they are empirically equivalent?

JHH: This actually leads to another kind of question. Most of you have heard of Chomsky's Universal Grammar. His notion was that it was so unlikely to have the ability to formulate a grammar that all examples were somehow 'wired in' as parameters and special values of a so-called Universal Grammar. This is something that is worth watching for in research in general. What Chomsky did was definitely a step forward: he introduced the notion of 'theory' into something that was stamp collecting before that. I mean people at the time of Linnaeus were collecting samples, and linguists were collecting all these examples like postage stamps, but they had no theory. In other words, it was simply what early exploration did.

Chomsky's Idea was that grammars were complicated enough that they somehow had to be instances wired in. That was a big advance. It really was a first attempt in a very real sense, producing something that was theoretical instead of stamp collecting. But it also soon became a huge barrier because you had no way to talk about learning or social interaction or any of these things that we consider very important in language. And so this happens more often than you might think where the advance then becomes an obstacle.

Jean-Pierre Changeux: You have introduced several levels of the notion of combinatorics. This is also a basic in Darwin's scheme. The viability through combinatorics. But then you have a mechanism which limits the viability or standardize the viability: this is selection. In the brain there are reward mechanisms which may be used to limit viability. But in your presentation you put reward at level 2 of consciousness. I think one of the missing aspects of linguistic is that even Chomsky does not take into consideration reward. In fact, there are rewards because at the end of the sentence which has meaning and sense there is a positive reward for the speaker. Why you did not talk about it?

JHH: Indeed, this is really this whole notion of fitness in a Darwinian sense. What I get involved in when I start thinking of that is there are genes in the chromosomes with as many as 10,000 copies of the same gene. What is the use of that? That seems a terrible waste of DNA. But if you think about it, it is very important because it lets the system explore, so to speak, without destroying the functions it already has. Now there is a lot more to it than that because the signaling mechanisms we did not use to know earlier, namely that signals can turn genes on and off that they can do all sorts of important actions. This is one of many examples that come to my mind. Or another example. Somehow we thought all of the bacteria in the gut were at the very least neutral. And now we know the notion of the microbiome and how important that is. But, again, we have very little theory about that. All we know is that it is at the present point of time very hard to go ahead with the notion of 'species' in bacteria. They exchange genetic material so rapidly and so often that the notion of 'species' becomes even difficult.

Jean-Pierre Changeux: How do you set the start point at a given level so that it would lead to an achievement.

JHH: Well, again my tendency is to think of the notion of hierarchies with exceptions. So I start out with something very simple like all animals move and then I realize that there are exceptions and these exceptions override the original notion. And that, in my terms, builds the so-called adaptive hierarchy.

So here is an example. "If it moves – freeze!" This turns out to be a pretty good rule for a frog because an awful lot of things that move are dangerous. But if the frog does that all the time, it has got some problems and it will never mate or it will never eat a fly because frogs and flies move. That is where the exception comes in and the exception overrides the earlier rule and it does not allow it to be executed. And if you can do some mathematics, you can produce a kind of a Sparse Matrix and so forth and so on. So you can do computation mathematics in that case which is sort of interesting.

BG: I am still interested in your view on how Nature builds up hierarchy. You used this nice example with the little bricks with which children play. And then you can calculate the probabilities of having more and more complex structures. But using this logic it would be an impossible task for Nature to build such a complex system as the human brain. What is your view on all this? Does Nature limit the almost infinite 'action space' so that the process determined by natural laws results in the evolution of the human brain?

JHH: I do not think this is a question of what Nature does. It is a question of how we observe Nature. I would really make the distinction here. I suggested earlier that if I want to make observations - and that is something which I as a human can do – I would need a 'control panel'.

Now let me say something not really silly but worth considering. Let us change the timescale tremendously and let us consider all the stars in our galaxy, moving about so forth and so on. If I change my timescale by a factor of what maybe a billion and if I were observing on that timescale, would it be appropriate to say on that timescale that our Galaxy is conscious?

Since consciousness is a matter in my terms of interactions, if I got this different timescale, could I describe it as the Galaxy on that timescale in the same terms that I now describe?

Per Roland: There is a book out now in which one physicist claims that everything that is in the universe can be described as mathematical structures. Would you agree with that?

JHH: Let me give you a measly answer. Largely, yes, and the reason I believe that is because the studies that I have made on the so-called Sparse Matrices seemed to give me a mechanism for describing the things in terms of the method of observation.

Per Roland: Good. Then someday our brain will be able to describe that as a set of mathematical structures.

JHH: I certainly hope so. I mean I hope at some point there comes a true theory of what we call complex adaptive systems. And you know that is a faith.

Roger Vergauwen: I think you are right in giving a measly answer because I would very much like to see the mathematics of causality which goes beyond correlation and to see what causality really is. We are not yet ready here...

JHH: When I see what I can do with Sparse Matrices, I see that this is not a matter of correlation but this is a matter of conditional action. And when I look at that, I'm hopeful.

BG: John, let me thank you for coming to Singapore for this event. We have really enjoyed your presence with us and for the intellectual food you have given us today. Thank you, John.

2 Synaptic Epigenesis and the Evolution of Higher Brain Functions*

Jean-Pierre Changeux

Département de Neurosciences, Institut Pasteur, Collège de France, Place Marcellin Berthelot, Paris, 25 Rue de Docteur Roux, Paris, France
changeux@pasteur.fr

The epigenesis theory of development can be traced back to William Harvey (1651), who stated, in contrast to contemporary preformation views, that the embryo arises by "the addition of parts budding out from one another." The word epigenesis was subsequently used by Conrad Waddington (Nature 150:563–565, 1942) to specify how genes might interact with their surroundings to produce a phenotype. This is also the meaning we adopted in our paper, Theory of the Epigenesis of Neuronal Networks by Selective Stabilization of Synapses (Changeux et al. Proc Nat Acad Sci U S A 70:2974–2978, 1973), according to which the environment affects the organization of connections in an evolving neuronal network through the stabilization or degeneration (pruning) of labile synapses associated with the state of activity of the network. This definition contrasts with the recent and more restricted sense of the status of DNA methylation and histone modification in a particular genomic region. The synapse selection theory was introduced to deal with two major features regarding the genetic evolution of the human brain: (1) the non-linear increase in the organizational complexity of the brain despite a nearly constant number of genes; and (2) the long postnatal period of brain maturation (ca. 15 years in humans), during which critical and reciprocal interactions take place between the brain and its physical, social and cultural environment. This theory will be evaluated and updated in the framework of the recent human/primate genome data, analysis of gene expression patterns during postnatal development, brain imaging of cultural pathways, such as those for language learning, and current views about the neural bases of higher brain func-tion, in particular the global neuronal workspace architectures for access to con-sciousness (see Dehaene and Changeux Neuron 70:200–227, 2011).

Introduction

The term 'epigenesis' (or 'epigenetics') should not be seen as applying only to molecular mechanisms of chromatin modification and the regulation of gene expression. Well before the term was hijacked by molecular biologists, we had applied it to a higher level of adaptation: the selection and stabilization of synaptic connections in the central nervous

* This chapter is reprinted with permission from the author and editor of *Epigenetics, Brain and Behavior*, P. Sassone-Corsi and Y. Christen (eds.), Research and Perspectives in Neurosciences II, (Springer Verlag 2012) DOI 10.1007/978-3-642-27913-3_2.

system by activity, through which the animal learns to adapt to its environment (Changeux *et al.*, 1973; Changeux and Danchin, 1976). The dramatic differences in structure and function between the brains of humans and lower mammals largely result from the high proportion of the connections in the human brain that are established during post-natal life. The continuation of the epigenetic mechanisms of synaptic selection throughout life are of particular significance in humans as they both underpin and are driven by social and cultural learning. Here I review the evidence for this type of epigenesis in the developing and adult nervous system.

One essential aspect of postnatal development in the human brain is the estab-lishment of long-range connections between different cortical areas, especially those linking the parieto-temporal-cingulate cortices with the prefrontal lobes, which are the centers for decision making, rational thinking and social interaction. According to our global neuronal workspace hypothesis (Dehaene *et al.*, 1998), these connections are a prerequisite for accessing consciousness. We are further testing the importance of their epigenetic stabilization in two animal model systems: genetically modified mice in which genes for a nicotinic receptor subunit have been deleted and quantitative evaluation of the expression profiles and activity dependence of 12,000 genes in the rat from embryo to adult. Some of these genes are involved in the regulation of chromatin modifications, providing a bridge between the synaptic and molecular levels of epigenetic regulation.

Defining Synaptic Epigenesis

The term epigenesis was first applied to the nervous system in the context of the selection and stabilization of synapses during development (Changeux *et al.*, 1973; Changeux and Danchin, 1976). The growth of axons towards their targets – the dendrites of target neurons in the central nervous system or muscle cells in the periphery – involves cell-surface recognition molecules, possibly ones unique to the specific category of connections. The axon terminals branch exuberantly at first but then are pruned back in response to neuronal activity, both intrinsic spontaneous neuron firing and that evoked by external inputs. Depending on the state of activity of the target neuron, some synapses are eliminated while others are strengthened and stabilized (Fig. 1). In post-natal life, an important part of the activity in the network results from inputs from the environment and so the epigenetic selection of synapses represents learning in the network as the organism is shaped to fit its environment. In this sense, learning can be considered as a Darwinian process, because it depends on elimination of the 'unfit' synapses.

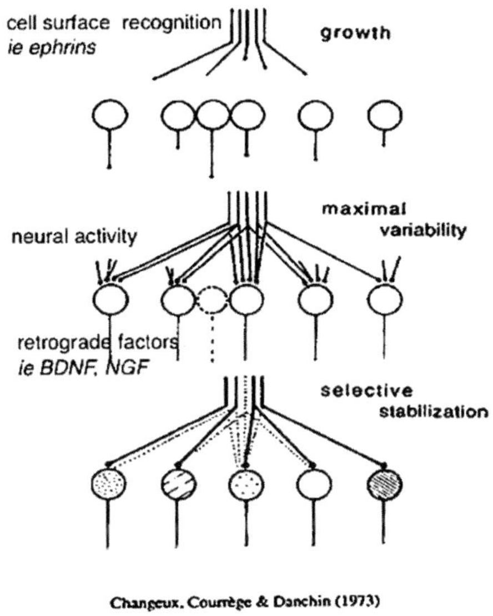

Fig. 1. Schematic representation of the hypothesis of epigenesis by selective stabilization of synapses. A nesting of many of such elementary steps occurs in the course of development. (from Changeux, 1985).

The word epigenetic was first used by William Harvey (1651), who, noting how complexity of form gradually emerges during embryogenesis, applied it to the description of how an embryo arises by "the addition of parts budding out from one another." In more modern times, the developmental biologist Conrad Waddington (1942) used the word to specify how genes interact with their sur-roundings to produce a phenotype. He conceived the concept of the 'epigenetic landscape' to illustrate how external events, some random, combine with inherited information coded in the genes to produce members of a species that, although recognizably related, have individual characteristics. His usage bridges the gap between synaptic epigenesis as defined above and the more molecularly oriented definition used in the introduction to this volume, i.e., mechanisms that permit variability beyond the Watson-Crick double helix.

One factor of considerable importance in discussing epigenetic mechanisms is that the brain is unique among organs in the specificity and number of its multiple connections between neurons (around 10^{15} in humans), a level of organization not found among, for example, the cells of the liver. Establishing and maintaining this huge connectivity requires a set of cellular processes and molecular mechanisms employed only in the nervous system.

Social and Cultural Evolution

Synaptic epigenesis is of particular significance in the context of the human brain because it enables social and cultural evolution (Changeux, 1985). Looking at the multiple levels of variability and their timescales within the human brain, we see, first, the variability of the genome, which underlies the biological evolution of the ancestors of *Homo sapiens* over millions of years. Next, on the ontogenetic or developmental level, is the epigenetic variability of neuronal networks and the connections that are established over days to years, depending on the species; beyond this, in humans, are the dynamics of thought, based on the variability of spontaneous/evoked neural activity and on the efficacy of synaptic connections, which operate in the 1–100 msec domain.

Finally, social and cultural evolution is associated with variable synaptic efficacy and the establishment of extracerebral memories in the form of spoken, written and pictorial material, with a time range of 100 msec to thousands of years. Spoken language and, perhaps even more significantly, writing are seminal innovations that distinguish humans from other primates; they drove the development of modern civilization and have probably also been central to the expansion of human mental capacities. Writing can be traced back to abstract cave drawings, dated around 30,000 BCE; clay counting tokens are known from Mesopotamia (9,000 BCE) and the first pictograms from Ur are from around 4,000 BCE. More important for my thesis, language and writing rely on epigenetic cultural transmission framed within a robust genetic envelope. The huge postnatal increase in the size of the human brain – the adult brain weighs five times that of the newborn infant and about 50 % of the adult brain's connections develop after birth (Huttenlocher and Dabholkar, 1997; Bourgeois, 1997) - offers the developing brain the opportunity for intense social and cultural interactions.

Paradoxically, the evolution of the genome has lagged well behind the increase in brain complexity during mammalian evolution (Venter *et al.*, 2001). The mouse, the rat and the monkey have approximately the same number of genes as a human (20,000-25,000). Yet the mouse has only

40 × 10^6 neurons, whereas the human brain contains in the range of 50–100 × 10^9. Gene sequences have not increased in complexity in parallel with the increase in complexity of the brain. Yet what happened? The explanation for this disparity, in my view, lies in a few genetic events that favored the prolonged and extensive post-natal increase in neuronal branching and synaptic connectivity in humans and its modulation by extended epigenetic responses to the environment.

Synaptic Selection and Stabilization

The extension of the post-natal period of development in humans has been essential for the genesis and internalization of culture, as well as for the acquisition and transmission of individual experience. In rats, the maximum synaptic density is reached within a few weeks after birth, whereas in humans it takes over three years. Moreover, rats show little loss of synapses after maximum density is reached, whereas in humans there is a steady decline until the total number stabilizes about the time of puberty (Huttenlocher and Dabholkar, 1997; Bourgeois, 1997; Petanjek *et al.*, 2011), reflecting the initial exuberance and later pruning of connections (cat and monkey show intermediate stages of this process as life span and infant dependency increase; Fig. 2). This major distinction between lower mammals and humans has to be borne in mind when using rats and mice as models for human psychiatric and neurological conditions. When *H. sapiens* appeared in Africa about 100,000 years ago, half the average life span of around 30 years would have been taken up with building the brain. And, of course, in contemporary humans, the process of synaptic refinement goes far beyond puberty: learning is lifelong (Petanjek *et al.*, 2011).

The decline in synaptic numbers during childhood reflects learning by selection. The initially exuberant connections are refined by activity in the network as some synapses are reinforced and others are eliminated (Fig. 1). Some early demonstrations of this process include work on motor neurons innervating muscle cells (Benoit and Changeux, 1975, 1978; O'Brien *et al.*, 1977; Henderson *et al.*, 1986; Gouzé *et al.*, 1983; Bourgeois *et al.*, 1986), the establishment of retinal inputs to the cat lateral geniculate body (Stretavan *et al.*, 1988); and studies in many other systems (Luo and O'Leary, 2005; Wu *et al.*, 2012; Kano and Hashimoto, 2011; Ko *et al.*, 2011).

These and many other studies have shown that, when neuronal activity is artificially modified, synaptic pruning is altered. In particular, at variance with the classical Lamarckist-constructivist scheme (Quartz and Sejnowski, 1997), blocking the activity maintains a high number of connections: it is activity that enhances synaptic elimi-nation (Benoit and Changeux, 1975, 1978; Stretavan *et al.*, 1988; Luo and O'Leary, 2005). As I have said in the past "to learn is to eliminate" (Changeux, 1985).

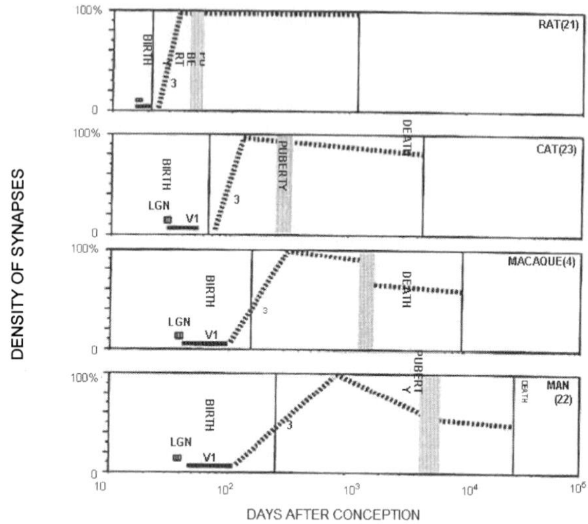

Fig. 2. Postnatal evolution of the total number of cortical synapses in different mammalian species. Note the significant decrease in the global envelope of synapses taking place before puberty in humans (from Changeux, 2004).

More recent work has revealed detailed mechanisms involved in synaptic plas-ticity, including processes of molecular selection by changes in the diffusion dynamics of receptors in the synaptic membrane while receptors maintain a stable density under the nerve ending (Triller and Choquet, 2008), and allosteric state transitions in the NMDA receptor trapping the diffusible D1 dopamine receptor that result in an increase in spines bearing dopamine receptors (Scott *et al.*, 2006), which is a plasticity phenomenon possibly altered in neuropsychiatric disorders.

Disruption of synapse selection and connectivity can also be seen in several human neurodevelopmental disorders. For instance, various mutations linked to autism are in genes that are involved in synapse formation/stabilization, such as NEUROLIGINS 3/4, NEUREXIN 1 and SHANK 3, which code for synaptic adhe-sion and stability proteins (Bourgeron, 2009). The dynamics of synapse stabilization is altered in Fragile X mental retardation by expanded CGG repeats in the FMR1 gene, which produces a protein that interferes with the Rac1 pathway and controls actin cytoskeleton dynamics (Mandel and Biancalana, 2004; Castets *et al.*, 2005). Changes in synaptic pruning have been associated with the onset of schizo-phrenia, a disease that has been linked to the susceptibility genes ERBB4, SLC1A3, RAPGEF4 and CIT28; the last is also involved in bipolar disorder (Karlsgodt *et al.*, 2008). Links with NEUREXIN 1, which is, as mentioned, involved in synapse formation/stabilization, have also been reported (Cook and Scherer, 2008).

The theory of the epigenesis of neuronal networks by selective stabilization of synapses (Changeux *et al.*, 1973) was introduced to account for the interactions that take place between the brain and its physical, social and cultural environment in the course of development; this theory therefore accounts for the variability in the brain's connectivity and in behavior between individuals, associated with the variability of the environment. Such an epigenetic variability of brain anatomy would be superimposed on that created by the variability of the genome. Another critical feature of the theory is that, conversely and unexpectedly, it may account for the constancy of some behaviors despite epigenetic variability. The same learning input may not stabilize the same connective patterns in different individuals but nevertheless result in the same behavior.

This idea was originally stated as the 'variability theorem' (Changeux *et al.*, 1973) that "different learning inputs may produce different connective organizations and neuronal functioning abilities, but the same behavioral abilities." This finding is particularly evident in the brains of genetically identical individuals that, contrary to expectation, do not show identical nerve organization. To give a simple example, the exact branching patterns of identified motor neurons in a parthenogenetic fish, *Poecilia formosa*, have been established by electron microscopy. This pattern was found to vary significantly not only between genetically identical individuals (identical twins) but also on the left and right sides of the same animal. Yet the fishes all swim the same way (Levinthal *et al.*, 1976). Thus, to some extent, the development of the fine details of the connectivity pattern includes a stochastic element - chance plays a part in determining exactly which synapses survive - yet the behavior may nevertheless remain constant between individuals. At a much higher level of com-plexity, humans with language areas located either in the left or right hemispheres, or in both, are indistinguishable by the way they speak or think! There is no contradiction between epigenetic "Darwinian" selection and the occurrence of behavioral universals.

One of the critical inputs that may contribute to synapse selection is reward (Thorndike, 1911; Hull, 1943; Skinner, 1981). Positive reward is signalled by neurons in the brain stem that release dopamine in the frontal cortex, whereas serotonin neurons signal negative reward, or punishment (Dehaene and Changeux, 1991, 2000). The evolution of connectivity through selection has been tested using a network simulation that can learn to do specific tasks when given simple positive and negative rewards (Gisiger *et al.*, 2005). Before learning, the connectivity in the network is diffuse and homogeneous and task completion is unsuccessful; after learning, the selected connections form a coherent and organized network that can complete tasks successfully. Further work should establish the actual contribution of reward to synapse selection in the course of development.

Epigenetics and Higher Brain Function

As already discussed, post-natal selection is essential for establishing the neuronal circuits serving culturally acquired behaviors such as writing and reading. By pains-takingly reconstructing the lesions in the brains of patients with various deficits, Dejerine (1901) was able to identify a variety of defects associated with learning written language. One such lesion caused an inability to read but left writing intact, a condition called pure alexia; the reverse lesion produced agraphia without alexia. These observations can be understood as evidence for separate epigenetic "cultural circuits" for reading and writing that are laid down in childhood.

More recently, the circuits involved in literacy have been examined using brain imaging. They confirm Dejerine's pionneering insight. These studies (Castro-Caldas *et al.*, 1998) took advantage of behavioral evidence of different phonological processing in illiterate vs literate subjects. During repetition of real words, the literate and illiterate groups performed similarly and activated similar areas of the brain. In contrast, illiterate subjects had more difficulty correctly repeating pseudowords and did not activate the same neural structures as literates. Compari-son of PET scans from illiterate and literate groups showed a considerable shift in activation. For instance, in a pseudowords – words contrast, activation in the literate group was stronger in the right frontal opercular – anterior insular region, left anterior cingulate, left lentiform nucleus and anterior thalamus/hypothalamus com-pared with the illiterate group (Castro-Caldas *et al.*, 1998; Carreiras *et al.*, 2009).

The connectivity used for reading and writing can thus be seen as an epigenetic appropriation of existing circuitry. Scans from ex-illiterates showed substantial similarity to those from literates, showing that the ability to acquire these cultural imprints persisted into adulthood (Dehaene *et al.*, 2010).

Among the cortical connections established in post-natal life are the long-range tracts between the frontal areas and other brain cortical areas (including sensory ones) that determine and organize action (see Pugliese *et al.*, 2009). Some years ago, we proposed that these long-range connections, by broadcasting signals to multiple brain areas, yield subjective experience (Dehaene *et al.*, 1998; Dehaene and Changeux, 2011). We termed this the 'global neuronal workspace' hypothesis: by allowing sensory inputs – seeing, hearing and so on – global access to many brain areas, the long-range connections provide a structural basis for the global experi-ence known as conscious access.

Long-range connections mostly originate from the pyramidal neurons in cortical layers II and III and are specially abundant in the prefrontal cortex (von Economo and Koskinas, 1925). Particularly important are the connections with the prefrontal areas, the part of the cortex involved in planning, decision making, thought and socializa-tion, that have evolved most dramatically between mice and humans (for a more detailed review of the global neuronal workspace hypothesis and its applications, see Changeux, 2006; Changeux and Lou, 2011; Dehaene and Changeux, 2011).

One question we are currently asking is whether these long-range connections are especially vulnerable to some pathologies. As mentioned above, the onset of schizophrenia has been linked to susceptibility genes coding for several proteins involved in synaptic pruning (Karlsgodt *et al.*, 2008; Cook and Scherer, 2008). Significantly, the long-range connections might be affected differentially by sus-ceptibility mutations that are known to affect synaptogenesis in general (Scott-Van Zeeland *et al.*, 2010). This vulnerability might result, for instance, from a very low nucleo-cytoplasmic ratio and/or changes in the long-distance transport of essential cellular components along the axons, which could explain the specificity of the schizophrenic phenotype as distinct from the mental retardation expected from a global deficit in synaptogenesis.

One way we are testing this vulnerability is by comparing the dendritic branching of pyramidal neurons in wild-type mice with animals lacking the β2-subunit of the nicotinic acetylcholine receptor (Ballesteros-Yáñez *et al.*, 2010). Loss of this subunit prevents the high-affinity binding of the neurotransmitter acetylcholine and, as a consequence, mice lacking the β2-subunit show a charac-teristic behavioral deficit: their exploratory drive, which is one of the most cogni-tive aspect of mouse behavior, is reduced, although their navigation abilities, a more automatic activity, are unaffected. Even though establishing a fair analogy between mouse behavior and human psychology may look far-fetched, it has been hypothesized that the mice might possibly be showing an alteration in elementary conscious access (see Avale *et al.*, 2011; reviewed in Changeux, 2006).

So far, we have not been able to examine the long-range projections but we have measured the complexity of the basal dendrites of 650 neurons from layer III in seven areas from the cortex of wild-type and β2−/− mice. In agreement with Elston's (2003) work on the monkey, the neurons in the wild-type mice show a gradient of complexity: those in anterior areas have longer dendrites, larger den-dritic fields and more spines. Such a complexity gradient may be interpreted in terms of the global neuronal workspace hypothesis as resulting from denser long-range connectivity originating from prefrontal areas. In contrast, the neurons in the knock-out mice are fairly uniform throughout the cortex, implying that the neurons in the frontal areas are not receiving as many inputs from the sensory areas as they do in the wild-type animals. In other words, the lack of nicotinic receptor activation seems to epigenetically enhance a selective loss of long-range connectivity.

These studies on mice may be relevant to a possible effect of chronic nicotine use on long-range connectivity. In humans, diffusion tensor imaging, which allows the meaurement of the location, orientation, and anisotropy of the white-matter tracts in the brain, has shown reduced integrity in the frontal white matter in people who are cocaine dependent or who abuse heroin. The same method has revealed that prenatal and adolescent exposure to tobacco smoke alters the development of the microstructure of the white matter, with increased fractional anisotropy in right and left frontal regions and in the genu of the corpus callosum (reviewed in Changeux and Lou, 2011). These observations suggest that nicotine may also act directly on white matter and there is electrophysiological evidence that supports a direct action of nicotine on axon conduction, possibly at the level of the node of Ranvier (reviewed in Changeux, 2010). Thus there is support for direct control of the global neuronal workspace by nicotine at the white matter level. This work further implies that drugs of abuse like nicotine may interfere with the functioning of the long-range cortical connections, so addicts may lose some conscious control of their actions.

Where Next?

We are turning back to the conventional tools of molecular genetics to map the expression patterns of genes involved in synaptic epigenesis throughout the life span of the rat. Using chip technology, the changes in expression of 12,000 genes in the cortex have been analyzed by computational methods at stages from embryonic day 16 through birth, puberty and adulthood to old age at post-natal day 90 (Tsigelny *et al.*, submitted). One dramatic change is at birth, when many genes active in the embryo are switched off and thousands of other genes become active, just as the animal goes through the most radical change in its environment that it is ever likely to encounter.

One fascinating aspect of this study is that some of the activated genes are involved in the regulation of chromatin modifications, which links the level of synaptic epigenesis that I have been discussing here back to the molecular mechanisms that are being detailed by other contributors to this volume.

Acknowledgments

The author thanks Yves Christen for his faithful support and Jennifer Altman for the careful transcription and editing of this paper.

References

Avale ME, Chabout J, Pons S, Serreau P, De Chaumont F, Olivo-Marin JC, Bourgeois JP, Maskos U, Changeux JP, Granon S (2011) Prefrontal nicotinic receptors control novel social interaction between mice. FASEB J 25:2145–2155.

Ballesteros-Yáñez I, Benavides-Piccione R, Bourgeois JP, Changeux JP, DeFelipe J (2010) Alterations of cortical pyramidal neurons in mice lacking high-affinity nicotinic receptors. Proc Natl Acad Sci U S A 107:11567–11572.

Benoit P, Changeux JP (1975) Consequences of tenotomy on the evolution of multiinnervation in developing rat soleus muscle. Brain Res 99:354–358.

Benoit P, Changeux JP (1978) Consequences of blocking the nerve with a local anaesthetic on the evolution of multiinnervation at the regenerating neuromuscular junction of the rat. Brain Res 149:89–96.

Bourgeois JP (1997) Synaptogenesis, heterochrony and epigenesis in the mammalian neocortex. Acta Paediatr Suppl 422:27–33.

Bourgeois JP, Toutant M, Gouzé JL, Changeux JP (1986) Effect of activity on the selective stabilization of the motor innervation of fast muscle posterior latissimus dorsi from chick embryo. Int J Dev Neurosci 4:415–429.

Bourgeron T (2009) A synaptic trek to autism. Curr Opin Neurobiol 19:231–234.

Carreiras M, Seghier ML, Baquero S, Estévez A, Lozano A, Devlin JT, Price CJ (2009) An anatomical signature for literacy. Nature 461:983–986.

Castets M, Schaeffer C, Bechara E, Schenck A, Khandjian EW, Luche S, Moine H, Rabilloud T, Mandel JL, Bardoni B (2005) FMRP interferes with the Rac1 pathway and controls actin cytoskeleton dynamics in murine fibroblasts. Hum Mol Genet 14:835–844.

Castro-Caldas A, Petersson KM, Reis A, Stone-Elander S, Ingvar M (1998) The illiterate brain. Learning to read and write during childhood influences the functional organization of the adult brain. Brain 121:1053–1063.

Changeux JP (1985) Neuronal man. Pantheon Books, New York.

Changeux JP (2004) The physiology of truth. Harvard University Press, Cambridge, MA.

Changeux JP (2006) The molecular biology of consciousness investigated with genetically modified mice. Philos Trans R Soc Lond B Biol Sci 361:2239–2259.

Changeux JP (2010) Nicotine addiction and nicotinic receptors: lessons from genetically modified mice. Nat Rev Neurosci 11:389–401.

Changeux JP, Danchin A (1976) Selective stabilisation of developing synapses as a mechanism for the specification of neuronal networks. Nature 264:705–712.

Changeux JP, Lou HC (2011) Emergent pharmacology of conscious experience: new perspectives in substance addiction. FASEB J 25:2098–2108.

Changeux JP, Courrège P, Danchin A (1973) A theory of the epigenesis of neuronal networks by selective stabilization of synapses. Proc Nat Acad Sci U S A 70:2974–2978.

Cook EH, Scherer SW (2008) Copy-number variations associated with neuropsychiatric conditions. Nature 455:919–923.

Dehaene S, Changeux JP (1991) The Wisconsin Card Sorting Test: theoretical analysis and modeling in a neuronal network. Cereb Cortex 1:62–79.

Dehaene S, Changeux JP (2000) Reward-dependent learning in neuronal networks for planning and decision making. Prog Brain Res 126:217–229.

Dehaene S, Changeux JP (2011) Experimental and theoretical approaches to conscious processing. Neuron 70:200–227.

Dehaene S, Kerszberg M, Changeux JP (1998) A neuronal model of a global workspace in effortful cognitive tasks. Proc Natl Acad Sci U S A 95:14529–14534.

Dehaene S, Pegado F, Braga LW, Ventura P, Nunes Filho G, Jobert A, Dehaene-Lambertz G, Kolinsky R, Morais J, Cohen L (2010) How learning to read changes the cortical networks for vision and language. Science 330:1359–1364.

Dejerine J (1901) Anatomie des centres nerveux (with Augusta Marie Dejerine-Klumpke). Rueff, Paris, 2 volumes.

Elston GN (2003) The pyramidal neuron in occipital, temporal and prefrontal cortex of the owl monkey (*Aotus trivirgatus*): regional specialization in cell structure. Eur J Neurosci 17:1313–1318.

Gisiger T, Kerszberg M, Changeux J-P (2005) Acquisition and performance of delayed-response tasks: a neural network model. Cereb Cortex 15:489–506.

Gouzé JL, Lasry JM, Changeux J-P (1983) Selective stabilization of muscle innervation during development: a mathematical model. Biol Cybern 46:207–215.

Harvey W (1651) Exercitationes de generatione animalium (On the generation of animals). Arnold Leers, The Hague.

Henderson CE, Benoit P, Huchet M, Guenet JL, Changeux JP (1986) Increase of neurite-promoting activity for spinal neurons in muscles of 'paralysé' mice and tenotomised rats. Brain Res 390:65–70.

Hull C (1943) Principles of behavior. Appleton-Century, Oxford.

Huttenlocher PR, Dabholkar AS (1997) Regional differences in synaptogenesis in human cerebral cortex. J Comp Neurol 387:167–178.

Kano M, Hashimoto K (2011) Activity-dependent maturation of climbing fiber to purkinje cell synapses during postnatal cerebellar development. Cerebellum. doi:10.1007/s12311-011-0337-3 (Epub ahead of print).

Karlsgodt KH, Sun D, Jimenez AM, Lutkenhoff ES, Willhite R, van Erp TG, Cannon TD (2008) Developmental disruptions in neural connectivity in the pathophysiology of schizophrenia. Dev Psychopathol 20:1297–1327.

Ko J, Soler-Llavina GJ, Fuccillo MV, Malenka RC, Su¨dhof TC (2011) Neuroligins/LRRTMs prevent activity and Ca2+/calmodulin-dependent synapse elimination in cultured neurons. J Cell Biol 194:323–334.

Levinthal F, Macagno E, Levinthal C (1976) Anatomy and development of identified cells in isogenic organisms. Cold Spring Harb Symp Quant Biol 40:321–331.

Luo L, O'Leary DD (2005) Axon retraction and degeneration in development and disease. Annu Rev Neurosci 28:127–156.

Mandel JL, Biancalana V (2004) Fragile X mental retardation syndrome: from pathogenesis to diagnostic issues. Growth Horm IGF Res 14(Suppl A):S158–S165.

O'Brien RA, Purves RD, Vrbová G (1977) Effect of activity on the elimination of multiple innervation in soleus muscles of rats. J Physiol 271:54P–55P.

Petanjek Z, Judaš M, Šimic G, Rasin MR, Uylings HB, Rakic P, Kostovic I (2011) Extraordinary neoteny of synaptic spines in the human prefrontal cortex. Proc Natl Acad Sci U S A 108:13281–13286.

Pugliese L, Catani M, Ameis S, Dell'Acqua F, Thiebaut de Schotten M, Murphy C, Robertson D, Deeley Q, Daly E, Murphy DG (2009) The anatomy of extended limbic pathways in Asperger syndrome: a preliminary diffusion tensor imaging tractography study. Neuroimage 47:427–434.

Quartz SR, Sejnowski TJ (1997) The neural basis of cognitive development: a constructivist manifesto. Behav Brain Sci 20:537–556, discussion 556–596.

Scott L, Zelenin S, Malmersjö S, Kowalewski JM, Markus EZ, Nairn AC, Greengard P, Brismar H, Aperia A (2006) Allosteric changes of the NMDA receptor trap diffusible dopamine 1 receptors in spines. Proc Natl Acad Sci U S A 103:762 767.

Scott-Van Zeeland AA, Abrahams BS, Alvarez-Retuerto AI, Sonnenblick LI, Rudie JD, Ghahremani D, Mumford JA, Poldrack RA, Dapretto M, Geschwind DH, Bookheimer SY (2010) Altered functional connectivity in frontal lobe circuits is associated with variation in the autism risk gene. CNTNAP2. Sci Transl Med 2:56ra80.

Skinner BF (1981) Selection by consequences. Science 213:501–504.

Stretavan DW, Shatz CJ, Stryker MP (1988) Modification of retinal ganglion cell axon morphology by prenatal infusion of tetrodotoxin. Nature 336:468–471.

Thorndike E (1911) Animal intelligence. Macmillan, New York (reprinted Thoemmes, Bristol 1999) Triller A, Choquet D (2008) New concepts in synaptic biology derived from single-molecule imaging. Neuron 59:359–374.

Tsigelny I, Kouznetsova V, Baitaluk M & Changeux J-P (submitted).

Venter JC, Adams MD, Myers EW, Li PW, Mural RJ, Sutton GG, Smith HO, Yandell M, Evans CA, Holt RA, Gocayne JD, Amanatides P, Ballew RM, Huson DH, Wortman JR, Zhang Q, Kodira CD, Zheng XH, Chen L, Skupski M, Subramanian G, Thomas PD, Zhang J, Gabor Miklos GL, Nelson C, Broder S, Clark AG, Nadeau J, McKusick VA, Zinder N, Levine AJ, Roberts RJ, Simon M, Slayman C, Hunkapiller M, Bolanos R, Delcher A, Dew I, Fasulo D, Flanigan M, Florea L, Halpern A, Hannenhalli S, Kravitz S, Levy S, Mobarry C, Reinert K, Remington K, Abu-Threideh J, Beasley E, Biddick K, Bonazzi V, Brandon R, Cargill M, Chandramouliswaran I, Charlab R, Chaturvedi K, Deng Z, Di Francesco V, Dunn P, Eilbeck K, Evangelista C, Gabrielian AE, Gan W, Ge W, Gong F, Gu Z, Guan P, Heiman TJ, Higgins ME, Ji RR, Ke Z, Ketchum KA, Lai Z, Lei Y, Li Z, Li J, Liang Y, Lin X, Lu F, Merkulov GV, Milshina N, Moore HM, Naik AK, Narayan VA, Neelam B, Nusskern D, Rusch DB, Salzberg S, Shao W, Shue B, Sun J, Wang Z, Wang A, Wang

X, Wang J, Wei M, Wides R, Xiao C, Yan C, Yao A, Ye J, Zhan M, Zhang W, Zhang H, Zhao Q, Zheng L, Zhong F, Zhong W, Zhu S, Zhao S, Gilbert D, Baumhueter S, Spier G, Carter C, Cravchik A, Woodage T, Ali F, An H, Awe A, Baldwin D, Baden H, Barnstead M, Barrow I, Beeson K, Busam D, Carver A, Center A, Cheng ML, Curry L, Danaher S, Davenport L, Desilets R, Dietz S, Dodson K, Doup L, Ferriera S, Garg N, Gluecksmann A, Hart B, Haynes J, Haynes C, Heiner C, Hladun S, Hostin D, Houck J, Howland T, Ibegwam C, Johnson J, Kalush F, Kline L, Koduru S, Love A, Mann F, May D, McCawley S, McIntosh T, McMullen I, Moy M, Moy L, Murphy B, Nelson K, Pfannkoch C, Pratts E, Puri V, Qureshi H, Reardon M, Rodriguez R, Rogers YH, Romblad D, Ruhfel B, Scott R, Sitter C, Smallwood M, Stewart E, Strong R, Suh E, Thomas R, Tint NN, Tse S, Vech C, Wang G, Wetter J, Williams S, Williams M, Windsor S, Winn-Deen E, Wolfe K, Zaveri J, Zaveri K, Abril JF, Guigo´ R, Campbell MJ, Sjolander KV, Karlak B, Kejariwal A, Mi H, Lazareva B, Hatton T, Narechania A, Diemer K, Muruganujan A, Guo N, Sato S, Bafna V, Istrail S, Lippert R, Schwartz R, Walenz B, Yooseph S, Allen D, Basu A, Baxendale J, Blick L, Caminha M, Carnes-Stine J, Caulk P, Chiang YH, Coyne M, Dahlke C, Mays A, Dombroski M, Donnelly M, Ely D, Esparham S, Fosler C, Gire H, Glanowski S, Glasser K, Glodek A, Gorokhov M, Graham K, Gropman B, Harris M, Heil J, Henderson S, Hoover J, Jennings D, Jordan C, Jordan J, Kasha J, Kagan L, Kraft C, Levitsky A, Lewis M, Liu X, Lopez J, Ma D, Majoros W, McDaniel J, Murphy S, Newman M, Nguyen T, Nguyen N, Nodell M, Pan S, Peck J, Peterson M, Rowe W, Sanders R, Scott J, Simpson M, Smith T, Sprague A, Stockwell T, Turner R, Venter E, Wang M, Wen M, Wu D, Wu M, Xia A, Zandieh A, Zhu X (2001) The sequence of the human genome. Science 291(5507):1304–1351.

Von Economo C, Koskinas GN (1925) Die cytoarchitektonik der hirnrinde des erwachsenen menschen. Springer, Vienna.

Waddington CH (1942) Canalization of development and the inheritance of acquired characters. Nature 150:563–565.

Wu X, Fu Y, Knott G, Lu J, Di Cristo G, Huang ZJ (2012) GABA signaling promotes synapse elimination and axon pruning in developing cortical inhibitory interneurons. J Neurosci 32:331–343.

3 East-West Differences and Implications for Cognitive Neuroscience

Stan Gielen

President, Dutch Science Foundation,
P.O. Box 93138, 2509 AC The Hague, Netherlands
S.Gielen@nwo.nl

Introduction

Much of the literature in Western Europe and the United States, suggests that East and West are, and always have been, separate entities with different cultural and scientific backgrounds. Irrespective of what is precisely meant by "East" and "West", no one will deny that the values that are used as guiding principles to organize society are very different in Western Europe and the United States on the one hand, and in Japan and China (as representatives for the Far East) on the other hand. Anyone from the West who has visited the East, and vice versa, will agree on the very different cultures and values in eastern and western societies. These differences not only relate to the basic values, like individual responsibility versus responsibility of society as a whole, honor, guilt, and happiness, but also to the history of eastern and western cultures. In western literature the notion prevails that the West has become the successful dominant part of the world due to its scientific rationality and its democratic principles. This view has been expressed, sometimes with a misplaced percept of superiority. According to this "Eurocentric" view, the Europeans spread over the world, conquering the far East and far West after Columbus discovered the Americas. However, this view has been challenged by several scholars, such as Hobson [2013] who presented convincing evidence, that there have been many interactions between Eastern and Western civilizations since 500 A.C. when North Africans and Muslims from the Middle East played a pioneering role in creating a global economy which connected the Far East and the West. Hobson gave an overview of the many interactions between the East and West and made the case that the rapid development of western civilization since the Middle Ages could not have taken place without the introduction of many discoveries in the East, such as gun powder, the production of steel and the use of coal for that purpose, and the compass for navigation. These discoveries were completely new for the West. The East and West have been in contact since many centuries with an exchange of ideas, knowledge, engineering skills and art. And yet, East and West always have been very different.

The Eurocentric view on the relationship between East and West may be wrong, the erroneous concept of the "superior West" illustrates once more the differences in attitude and cultural perspective since the Middle Ages. East and West have developed in very different directions regarding values as guiding principles for society and happiness. Yet, long time ago, both East and West shared many views on happiness and a good life. Both the Buddha in the East, as well as Socrates and Seneca in the West considered happiness as a state of mind, which could be achieved by active pursuit and interference with events in the environment and by contemplation, reflection and introspection. Wisdom and knowledge about the world and about oneself were considered by philosophers and many politicians as more important than wealth. Since then, much has changed. In the West the idea now prevails that individuals are responsible for a large part for their own success and happiness. The emphasis on the individual to create favorable conditions for happiness is dominant in the West, culminating in the idea of the American Dream, where everyone can achieve the near impossible.

In this chapter we will focus on the relationship between happiness and what subjects can do to improve happiness and a good life at the one hand and neuroscience at the other hand. Meditation is a familiar aspect to make a good life in the East and gradually more people in the West participate in meditation groups to reduce stress, to improve the ability to concentrate on what really matters without distraction by irrelevant issues, and to develop a more compassionate behavior to other people. What happens in the brain when subjects pay attention to objects in the environment and to other people and when they make decisions (or abstain from making decisions)? And what happens to the brain when subjects meditate? What is the impact of meditation on brain function and brain connectivity? Is there a scientific platform, which allows us to understand what it means to be happy and to have a good life and how we can work on that from a neuroscientific approach.

These questions cannot be all satisfactorily answered in one book, let alone in one chapter. Happiness and "a good life" are broad concepts which are hard to define and the definition may be different in different parts of the world. Much psychological, sociological and neuroscience research has been done and major questions are unanswered yet. In this chapter we will provide an overview of recent insights and developments, with proper references for further reading. An excellent book, which deals with happiness and a good life from a social psychological point of view, is the book "In search of happiness, the psychology of a good life" by Dijksterhuis [2015], which unfortunately is (not yet) available in English. Another useful book on happiness is by McMahon [2006], which gives an excellent overview from a historical perspective, starting with the classical views in ancient Greece up to the contemporary view on or, if one wishes, obsession with happiness.

Historical Consideration Regarding a "Good Life" in East and West

A short historical perspective on happiness and a good life

In prehistory, life was hard for people living those days, but the strategy for making a good life was relatively simple: make sure to please the good gods and avoid to annoy the bad gods. If evil fell upon you, it was because you had done something wrong by making the gods angry, or because a bad god decided to make life hard on you. Another possibility was that God was testing you, like in the Book of Job in the Old Testament, where God, challenged by the devil, tested Job by taking all his goods, expelling him from his house and village and by killing all his beloved ones.

After the introduction of Christianity, especially after Augustine (354-430 AC), the main purpose of life in the West was not to make a happy life, but was to serve God, mainly by obeying his rules and by doing well to others. According to the Catholic church those days, suffering on earth was unavoidable, but the key for a good life was to serve God and by doing so to deserve a seat in heaven for eternity. Yet, this doctrine was not completely satisfactory, since it was hard to perceive why a good and almighty God might allow people to act against God's will and to do evil things to other people. This raised the discussion about predestination after Luther in the 16th and 17th centuries in Western Europe, but in short, the main aim remained for a long time to live on earth in the hope for a good life after death.

An attempt to deal with the question how the notion of a good and almighty God could be reconciled with the fact of crimes and disaster in society was made by the German philosopher and mathematician

Leibniz who argued that this world was the best of all possible worlds that God could create. Yet, this did not stop wondering why a good God could create a world full of innocent suffering. This became a major topic after the Lisbon earthquake in 1755 which destroyed the city of Lisbon and killed several thousand of its inhabitants. This event shook the Enlightment all the way to East Prussia where Immanuel Kant, at that time an unknown minor scholar, wrote three essays in the Köningsberg newspaper on the nature of earthquakes. Later Voltaire and Rousseau wrote several manuscripts on this topic. In later years Kant argued that God, along with many other subjects of classical metaphysics, exceeded the limits of human knowledge (see Neiman [2002] for an excellent overview on the topic of evil in modern thought). Obviously, the argument that God and his intentions with mankind exceed the limits of human knowledge eliminates any further discussion about God's role in explaining the innocent suffering in society.

After decades of attempts to explain innocent suffering without questioning the role of God, the Enlightment started the discussion about the role of God and about the courage to think for oneself, or in other words, the courage to take responsibility for the world in which we live. The changing emphasis on happiness during this life became prominent in the Declaration of Independence by Thomas Jefferson in 1776 and in the principles of the French Revolution at the end of the 18th century. Since then the emphasis gradually shifted to the wish of individual happiness in this life and the idea that each person is in control of his own life, and thereby is able to contribute to his own fortune and happiness. This is best illustrated by the notion of the "American Dream", which says that all people have the same rights and that everyone can achieve his/her goals, if one just works hard enough to pursue these goals.

Genetic and environmental aspects, relevant for a "good life"

If we speak about civilizations and communities with particular values, we speak about human subjects and their interactions, which together define a community or society. The behavioral repertoire of human beings is the result of genetic and environmental components, which affect the neuronal activity and neuronal connectivity and thereby shape the behavior and thoughts of individual subjects. The neuronal architecture depends on genetic factors, but due to plasticity of the brain it is also affected by the environment and by interactions between subjects, and therefore, by cultural values and by environmental aspects, such as climate, geographic conditions and the availability of suitable land for agriculture or hunting. If we have to spend much time to collect food, there is little time left for introspection, reflection and art. A Mediterranean climate does require less time to build shelter and a home than in cold and rainy parts of the Northern Europe. This does not only affect the living conditions, it also affects the social interactions between people and thereby the development of the brain. This raises the question as to whether and to what extent the different cultural, political and scientific environment including language, life style and social environment may affect the behavior and perceived well-being of people, and the question to what extent differences in genetic background are involved. Most studies assume that genetic factors only play a modest role in shaping society. In the last century, a large part of the immigrants entering the west coast of the USA had an Asian background. Although there will definitely be some genetic differences, the majority of Asian immigrants adapted quite well and successfully to the USA life style and were able to develop a "good life". This suggests that people adapt to new living conditions and that Nurture is an important factor which shapes the behavioral repertoire of human subjects and thereby also contributes to the feeling of well-being and happiness.

Studies on happiness have shown that human subjects are able to make a happy life, even in miserable conditions, as long as their living conditions are more or less stable. This excludes conditions of war, famine and other natural disasters. People in general adapt within several months to unexpected living conditions to make the best out of it. A study by Brickman *et al.* [1978] followed three groups of subjects. One group had won more than $50,000 in a lottery (one third even more than 1 million dollars). A second group of subjects had developed a hemiplegia due to accidents or diseases, and then there was a control group. Although winning a lottery or becoming handicapped affected their rating for happiness at or right after the event, it hardly affected their expectations on happiness for the long term. Surprisingly, after about 6 months, the ratings for perceived happiness did not differ significantly any more among groups. Another study [Biswas-Diener and Diener, 2001] followed a large number of people in the slums of Kolkata (former Calcutta, India). Although life is miserable in these slums, at least according to most western standards, the average satisfaction with their life was rated as 2.23 on a scale between 1 (negative) and 3 (positive).

Therefore, external circumstances certainly affect the subjective feeling of a “good life”, but may be less dominant than generally thought.

We all know that the genetic information determines to a large part the personal traits, the cognitive skills and many other physical, psychological, and social properties of a person. Not the least are the architecture of the brain and the connections between different parts of the brain the result of the information in the human genome. On the other hand we also know that human activity shapes the brain. If you want to become a good piano player, you have to practice. By practicing, neuronal connections are modified so as to adjust and to optimize brain connectivity and brain function for this task. This raises the question how do subjects adapt to new circumstances? What happens to them, not only when fortune or bad luck comes to them, but also when they develop a stable happy life by introspection, reflection or by a successful pursuit for happiness. What happens in the brain when people feel happy and what brain properties ensure that people feel happy in general? Can we provide a scientific framework, which explains why people feel happy, even in dark and miserable circumstances, and how can we use this information to help people to become happy?

It is obvious that both genetic factors, as well as environmental aspects contribute to the feeling of happiness and a good life. On top of that, subjects can actively pursue happiness by modifying living conditions. Since feeling good and active pursuit to feel good both are reflected in brain activity [Wise, 2002], the question comes up to what extent and in which way the brain can make decisions to actively seek for satisfactory rewards and happiness. In this chapter we will focus on two questions relating brain activity and well-being. First we will give an overview of recent developments in neuroscience, which explain how bottom-up sensory information may affect higher cognitive processes and how top-down cognitive processes may selectively modulate sensory information. After that we will describe how subjects can affect brain activity and connectivity by active behavior, such as meditation. Since all emotions and opinions find their roots in brain activity, we will explore how differences in living in the East and West are reflected in activity of the brain and how approaches from the East, such as (mindfulness) meditation affect brain activity and thereby affect human behavior.

Learning, Adaptation and Self-Organization in the Human Brain

Neuronal information coding

The human brain consists of about 10^{11} nerve cells, also called "neurons". Each neuron sends its signals to other neurons by nerve fibers, called axons. These axons branch out to many other neurons, such that on average each neuron is connected to about a thousand other neurons. The output of a neuron is a series of electrical pulses each with a duration of about 1 millisecond and each electrical pulse serves as input to about thousand (on average) other neurons. In general, a sufficiently large input from many input neurons in a relatively short time interval (say 10-100 ms) is required to activate the output neuron and to elicit an electrical pulse in the output neuron.

The effective input from a neuron to another neuron depends on the connection strength, which is not fixed but flexible. The connection strength changes in time, proportional to the correlation between firing of the input neuron and the output neuron. The basic mechanism is that the connection strength between neuron *a* and a neuron *b*, which receives input from neuron *a*, is proportional to the correlation in activity of the input and output neurons. If neuron *b* sends an output signal right after arrival of input from *a*, the connection strength between neurons *a* and *b* becomes stronger. When the output neuron *b* on average fires before input from *a* arrives, this means that it is the input from other neurons (not neuron *a*) which activates neuron *b*, and then the connection strength between neurons *a* and *b* becomes weaker.

Neurons send information as a sequence of electrical pulses, which propagate along the axons. The information in the neuronal signal is encoded in the rate of pulses (typically in the range between 1 to 100 pulses/s) and in the amount of synchrony of the pulses in a population of neurons. If the pulses in a population of neurons are generated independently, the pulses of neurons in the population appear in random order. However, if the neurons synchronize their pulses, the pulses of the population of neurons reveal rhythmic activity. The frequency of these rhythms may vary and appears to cluster in several frequency bands, such as the frequency range 3-7 Hz (called theta-band), 8-13 Hz (called alpha-band), 13-30 Hz (called beta-band), 30-80 Hz (gamma band). Each of these rhythms has a specific function as we will explain later.

Neuronal networks and functional connectivity

Since the early stages of brain research, the brain has been subdivided in anatomical units (such as hippocampus, thalamus, cortex, cerebellum, each with its own characteristic anatomical structure) and in functional units, such as visual cortex, auditory cortex, and motor cortex. The subdivision in anatomical units makes sense, since a different anatomical architecture presumably also implies a different functionality. The distinction in functional units also makes sense. For example, there is a region in the posterior part of cortex, which becomes active mainly after presentation of visual stimuli. Cells in this brain region respond to very specific features in the visual stimulus. Similarly, there are regions exclusively active after presentation of auditory stimuli (auditory cortex), after tactile stimulation (somatosensory cortex) and just before movements (motor cortex). Much of our current knowledge of cognitive brain function has come from this modular paradigm, in which brain areas are postulated to act as independent processors for specific complex cognitive functions. Recent findings, however, suggest that this paradigm has serious limitations. For example, there are hardly any tasks, if at all, in which visual cortex is active in complete isolation. Visual cortex is typically active when reading a book, driving a car, or looking for a beer in the refrigerator. In all these conditions, visual cortex is active as part of a complex activity which involves many more brain areas, like storing information in memory when reading a book, steering your car along the road or making head and eye movements to explore the content of the refrigerator. In all these conditions, visual cortex is part of a network of brain regions, and this network changes depending on the task or intention of the person. This is very similar to the architecture of a modern computer. Everyone is familiar with the hard disk (to store information), the Central Processing Unit (CPU) for all computations, the dynamic random access memory (to make information accessible to the CPU), and the video card for visual display of information. A computer is not complete (and in fact useless) without each of these units. However, these units, each with their own functionality, are active in various combinations all the time, depending on the specific processing task.

Because each part of the brain participates in flexible networks, the information exchange is flexible and task-dependent, which explains why even the functions of primary sensory areas of the cerebral cortex, once thought to be pinnacles of modularity, are being redefined by recent evidence of cross-modal interactions. A new paradigm in cognitive neuroscience has emerged that moves beyond the simplistic mapping of cognitive constructs onto individual brain areas and emphasizes instead the conjoint function of brain areas working together as large-scale functional networks.

Functional brain networks and neuronal oscillations

The human brain is a complex processing device which adapts to the environment. A good example is the perception of objects in depth. Because the two eyes have a slightly different position, the images of the environment on the retinas are slightly different. This disparity encodes information about direction and distance of objects in the environment. During childhood, the connections between neurons develop in such a way that neurons in visual cortex become responsive to depth cues in the visual stimulus. However, if this binocular information is not available (such as in amblyopia), neurons will never respond to depth cues. This is an example of changes in connectivity at a long time scale.

However, changes in the functional architecture are also found at a time scale of milliseconds, such as in the case of attention. This is illustrated in Fig. 1 which shows typical brain areas active in three different tasks. Attention is characterized by three different mechanisms. The alerting (sustained attention or vigilance) network is defined as achieving and maintaining an alert state. Sustained attention, vigilance and alertness define the ability to increase and maintain response readiness in preparation for an impending stimulus. This is important if one aims to be alert for specific new events and if distractors have to be ignored. Therefore, the alerting network involves activation or increased excitability of networks that are involved in processing expected stimuli, and inhibition or decreased excitation of brain areas that are not relevant for the expected stimuli. Another network is the orienting attention network. Orienting is the ability to select specific information from among multiple sensory stimuli. Orienting attention can be overt or covert (for example, with or without eye movements). A typical example of a combination of overt and covert attention is when driving a car, which requires overt attention on the curvature of the road and any other cars on the road which need your attention to avoid collisions or to get rid of the road. However, covert attention is required for children playing on the sidewalks, who might unexpectedly chase for toys on the roadway. Finally, there is the executive attention, which involves top-down control or the monitoring of conflict between processing in different neural areas related to planning or decision making, error detection, new or not well-learned conditions judged to be difficult or dangerous, regulation of thoughts and feelings. For an overview, see Raz and Buhle [2006].

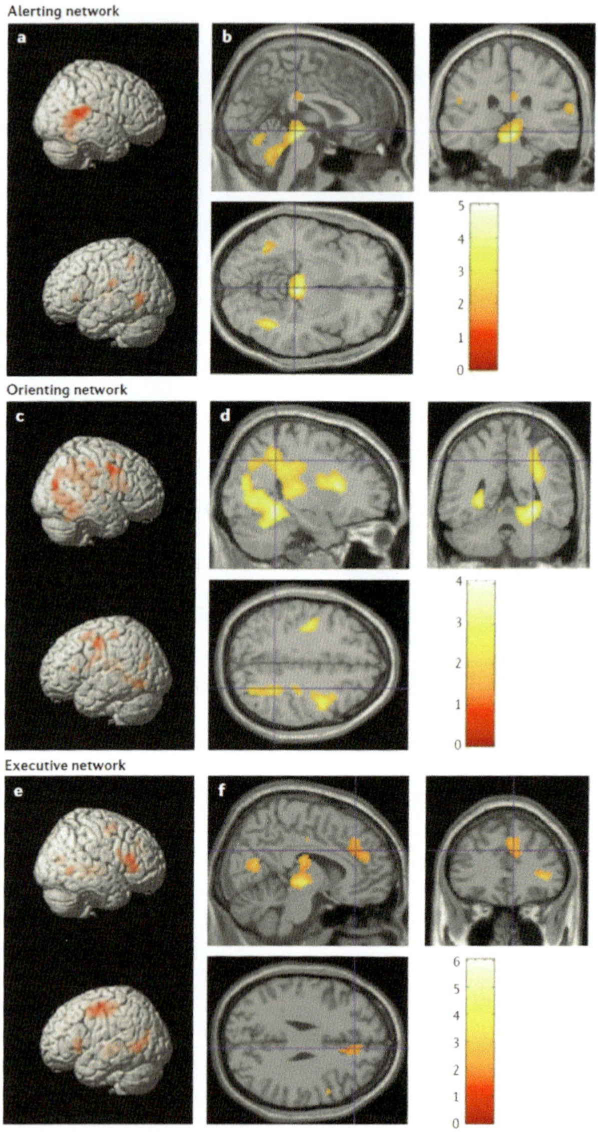

Fig. 1. The panels show cross-sectional views of the three attentional networks: the alerting network with thalamic activation (**a,b**), the orienting network shows parietal activation (**c,d**), and the conflict network shows anterior cingulated cortex activation (**e,f**). The color bar shows fMRI signal level (Z-scores) above the 0.05 significance threshold. (Copied with permission from Raz and Buhle, 2006).

Figure 1 shows the activity of brain areas measured by functional Magnetic Resonance Imaging (fMRI) for the three attentional tasks. It illustrates that quite different brain areas are active in these tasks and these networks can be created or annihilated within tenths of milliseconds. They are shaped by both bottom-up sensory information as well as top-down cognitive processes. The latter modulate or gate the sensory information processing and thereby enable or disable particular brain areas and define the functional network.

What does this tell us about decision making by human subjects? How do bottom-up and top-down information interact? This question has been the topic of many studies. In daily life, there is an abundance of objects in the environment which provide visual, auditory and tactile input to the brain. Because not all objects are of interest, we focus our attention on objects of interest and suppress information from irrelevant objects. The latter is achieved by top-down generated oscillations in the alpha-band (called alpha rhythm) induced in that part of the brain which should not be involved in neuronal information processing. Oscillatory activity in the alpha-band has been shown to be related to inhibition of distraction. An increase in alpha band activity is correlated with a decrease in neuronal excitability [Romei *et al.*, 2008; Haegens *et al.*, 2011; Jensen *et al.*, 2012]. Consequently, it has been proposed that alpha band activity serves to route information to downstream regions by inhibiting neuronal processing in task-irrelevant regions.

This is illustrated in Fig. 2 which shows the power of electrical (EEG) activity measured with surface electrodes on the skull in a task where subjects have to pay attention to visual objects in a particular part of visual space which involves neuronal processing in the right visual cortex. In this experiment the lower two panels show an increase in power near 10 Hz (i.e. in the alpha band) in the left part of visual cortex and a decrease of power in the alpha band for the right part of visual cortex. These changes in alpha-band activity start about 300 milliseconds after presentation of a cue, which signals the upcoming presentation of objects on a screen in front of the subject. The upper part of Fig. 2 shows the distribution of alpha-band activity, revealing a clear topology and lateralisation in the alpha-band activity.

The functional significance of the alpha-band activity becomes clear when different visual stimuli are presented and when subjects had to respond in a different way to each visual stimulus. Typically, one uses a task where subjects make errors easily, either because the task is very complex or very boring. Mazaheri and Jensen [2009] used a quite boring task, where a cue was presented, followed by a digit in the range from 0 to 9. The subject was instructed to push a button after presentation of the digit, except when the digit was the digit "5". Because of the quite boring nature of the experimental condition, the amount of alpha activity varies and consequently, the gating of irrelevant visual information was modulated, resulting in error responses where subjects also pushed the button when the digit "5" appeared. Errors appeared to be made particularly, when lateralization of the alpha-band activity was less pronounced and when the power in the alpha-band was small in visual cortex. Mazaheri *et al.* [2009] found a significant correlation between the decrease in alpha-band power and the probability of an erroneous response. Based on the decrease of alpha-power, they were able to predict quite accurately when subjects would make errors in their responses to the stimuli. All this implies that top-down processes selectively gate relevant and irrelevant information.

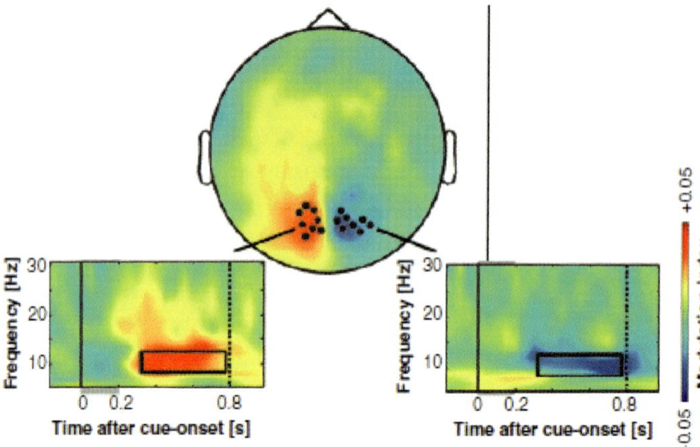

Fig. 2. The hemispheric lateralization is thought to reflect the allocation of attentional resources: the decrease of activity in the alpha band coincides with the engagement of task-relevant areas, whereas the increase in activity in the alpha band coincides with functional inhibition. At time zero a cue is presented followed by a visual stimulus, which requires visual processing in the right visual cortex. Lower panels show the frequency distribution of the EEG activity in visual cortex as a function of time. The upper panel shows the distribution of alpha power across the skull. (Copied with permission from Jensen *et al.* [2012]).

The next question then is: how is this top-down modulation of sensory activity achieved? What modulates the alpha activity in visual cortex? This question is partly answered by studying the activity in prefrontal cortex. It is well known that prefrontal cortex is involved in decision making and in the control of selective attention. It appears that activity in prefrontal cortex in the theta-band (range 3-7 Hz) modulates alpha activity in visual cortex [Cavanagh and Frank, 2014]. If the theta-band activity in prefrontal cortex after error trials is compared to that after successful trials, activity in the theta-band appears to be much larger in the former condition after the error response (see Fig. 3) and the theta-activity in prefrontal cortex modulates the alpha activity to prevent errors next time (not shown). The prefrontal cortex can be considered as the conductor of the brain, much like the conductor in an orchestra where the conductor decides when instruments set in and at what rhythm and intensity. The conclusion of these results is that the state of the brain determines how incoming stimuli are processed and how subjects respond.

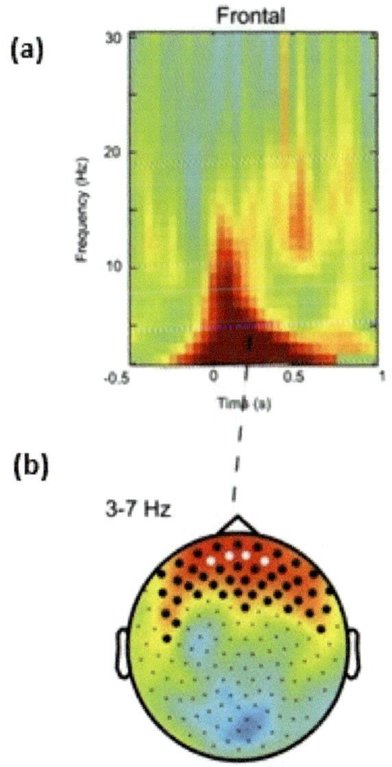

Fig. 3. (a) Grand average of the difference time-frequency representations (Error trials – correct trials) of representative frontal sensors (sensors marked in white) in a task where subjects had to press a key after appearance of a digit in the range 0-9, except when the digit was the digit "5". The button press occurred at t = 0 s. (b) Grand average of the topography of activity in the theta band (3–7 Hz). (Copied with permission from Mazaheri *et al.* [2009]).

How cognitive states affect brain activity: studies on mindfulness

Meditation is typically associated with the East as a way to explore the mind, to explore one's conscious thoughts and to strive for equanimity by transforming our mind from negative to positive, from disturbed to peaceful, from unhappy to happy. Overcoming a negative mind set and cultivating constructive thoughts is the purpose of the transforming meditations found in the Buddhist tradition.

In the past decades, meditation has also become popular in the West as a way to deal with stress, to improve concentration, to avoid negative thoughts and to find a peace of mind. One of the pioneers in the West was Jon Kabat-Zinn, who ventilated the powerful and beneficial effects of mindfulness meditation. He also used mindfulness meditation as a therapy to reduce stress (Mindfulness-Based Stress Reduction or MBSR), which has led to a large increase in clinical applications and empirical research on mindfulness-meditation-based interventions, such as MBSR. The mindfulness-meditation-based practices have proven to be effective in reducing the clinical symptoms in a considerable number of psychological, psychosomatic, and emotional disturbances [Baer, 2003; van den Hurk *et al.*, 2010; Kabat-Zinn, 2003; Chiesa *et al.*, 2011]. His work has triggered much research on the effect of mindfulness meditation and on the neurophysiological mechanisms that are related to meditation.

Despite the fact that a growing body of scientific literature about the clinical applications of mindfulness meditation seems to reveal promising results of its effectiveness, surprisingly few studies have addressed the neuropsychology and neurophysiology related to mindfulness meditation, and very little is known about the mechanism(s) by which mindfulness meditation exerts its effect(s). As mindfulness meditation has been described as "a particular way to pay attention" [Kabat-Zinn, 2003], a putative candidate mechanism for its effect(s) is a modification in attentional processing. More specifically, several studies have reported that mindfulness meditation leads to improvement of the self-regulation of attention. In recent pioneering studies, Jha *et al.* [2007] and van den Hurk *et al.* [2010] used the attention network test to examine changes in attentional processing induced by mindfulness meditation. They performed a longitudinal study with three groups: a group of meditators who have much experience during retreats ("retreat group"), a group who participated in MBSR, and a control group. These authors found a significantly better attention network in the retreat group, both in reaction time (RT) and in error score (ES) data, where ES was defined as the percentage of incorrect responses. Overall, the picture that emerges from the literature is that early phases of mindfulness training, which are more concerned with the development of focused attention, could be associated with significant improvements in selective and executive attention whereas the following phases, which are characterized by an open monitoring of internal and external stimuli, can be mainly associated with improved unfocused sustained attention abilities. Additionally, subjects who participate in mindfulness meditation can enhance working memory capacity and some executive functions.

The state of mindfulness has often been described as a state of "presence of mind" which concerns a clear awareness of one's inner and outer worlds, including thoughts, sensations, emotions, actions or surroundings as they exist at any given moment. Hence it may not be surprising that mindful awareness and mindfulness meditation have an effect on attentional processes in the brain and that these effects become visible in behavioral tasks and neuronal activity related to attention. Modern neuroimaging techniques, such as functional MRI (fMRI) allow the identification of functional networks in the brain.

Modern neuroimaging studies have revealed the neuronal mechanisms which underlie the behavioral changes induced by meditation, which have been described above. Kilpatrick *et al.* [2011] have shown that mindfulness meditation increases functional connectivity within auditory and visual networks and increases functional connectivity between auditory cortex and areas associated with attentional and self-referential processes. Changes in functional connectivity were significant already after 8 weeks of mindfulness meditation training, reflecting a more consistent attentional focus, enhanced sensory processing, and reflective awareness of sensory experience.

In a recent study Luders *et al.* [2011] investigated the connectivity in a well-matched sample of long-term meditators and controls using diffusion tensor imaging (DTI). DTI is a technique to investigate white matter fiber characteristics. They reported a pronounced structural connectivity in meditators compared to controls throughout the entire brain. While cross-sectional studies represent a good starting point for elucidating possible links between meditation and white matter fiber characteristics, more longitudinal studies will be necessary to determine the relative contribution of nature and nurture to enhanced structural connectivity in long-term meditators.

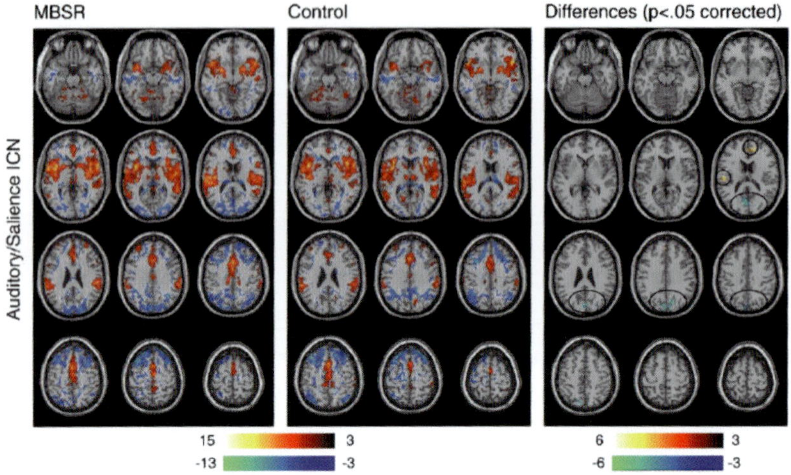

Fig. 4. Single group maps of the auditory/salience ICN for MBSR subjects (left panel) and wait list controls subjects (middle panel) are presented. In the right panel, significant group differences are shown; red indicates areas of significantly increased functional connectivity while blue indicates areas of greater anti-correlation with the auditory/salience ICN in MBSR subjects compared to wait list controls. (Copied with permission from Kilpatrick *et al.* [2011]).

Summary

The results of psychological, clinical, and neurophysiological studies have convincingly shown that mindfulness meditation does have a positive effect on well-being. It reduces stress and it helps people to deal with unpleasant situations, such as disease or death. Moreover, meditation leads to improved attention and concentration and it does so already after about 8 weeks of training. These changes in behavior are reflected by changes in brain activity and connectivity. Both bottom-up sensory processing as well as top-down cognitive control are affected by attention and mindfulness meditation. These effects are evident in behavioral studies and in neurophysiological/anatomical studies, which have revealed changes in neuronal activity and connectivity due to mindfulness meditation. These results show that practice makes a large contribution to changes in behavior and brain activity.

These neurophysiological results are consistent with recent sociological results of studies on happiness [Dijksterhuis, 2015], which suggest that happiness is by 40% the result of genetically encoded properties, which are common to people in the East and West. Environmental contributions and active participation by subjects explain

10% and 50%, respectively, indicating that Nurture is approximately equally important as Nature. Obviously, these data pertain to the average person in western society. If someone lives in a region with war and famine, these numbers will be different.

This may be good news, as it indicates that subjects are, to some extent, in control in being happy and making a good life. Although there are differences between the lifestyle in the East and West, subjects are free to choose the style that fits best to them in making a good life, and by doing so "shape" their brain for a happy life.

References

Baer, R. A. (2003). Mindfulness training as a clinical intervention: A conceptual and empirical review. *Clin. Psychol.: Science and Practice*, 10, pp. 125-143.

Biswas-Diener, R. and Diener, E. (2001). Making the best of a bad situation: satisfaction in the slums of Calcutta. *Social Indicators Research*, 55, pp. 329-352.

Brickman, P., Coates, D. and Janoff-Bullman, R. (1978). Lottery winners and accident victims: Is happiness relative? *Journal of Personality and Social Psychology* 36, pp. 917-927.

Cavanagh, J. F. and Frank, M. J. (2014). Frontal theta as a mechanism for cognitive control, *Trends Cogn. Sciences*, 18, pp. 414-421.

Chiesa, A., Calati, R. and Serretti, A. (2011). Does mindfulness training improve cognitive abilities? A systematic review of neuropsychological findings, *Clin. Psychol. Rev.* 31, pp. 449-464.

Dijksterhuis, A. (2015). *Op naar geluk. De psychology van een fijn leven*. (Prometheus, Netherlands).

Haegens, S., Nacher, V., Luna, R., Romo, R. and Jensen, O. (2011). alpha-oscillations in the monkey sensorimotor network influence discrimination performance by rhythmical inhibition of neuronal spiking, *Proc. Natl. Acad. Sci. USA*, 108, pp. 10377-10382.

Hobson, J. M. (2013). *The eastern origins of western civilization*. 10th Ed. (Cambridge University Press, UK).

Jensen, O., Bonnefond, M. and VanRullen, R. (2012) An oscillatory mechanism for prioritizing salient unattended stimuli, *Trends Cogn. Sciences*, 16, pp. 200-206.

Jensen, O. and Mazaheri, A. (2010). Shaping functional architecture by oscillatory alpha activity: gating by inhibition, *Front. Hum. Neurosci.* 4:186, doi: 10.3389/fnhum.2010.00186.

Jha, A. P., Krompinger, J. and Baime, M. J. (2007). Mindfulness training modifies subsystems of attention. *Cogn. Aff. & Behav. Neurosci.*, 7(2), pp. 109-119.

Kabat-Zinn, J. (2003). Mindfulness based interventions in context: Past, present, and future. *Clin. Psychol.: Science and Practice*, 10, pp. 144-156.

Kilpatrick, L. A., Suyenobu, B. Y., Smith, S. R., Bueller, J. A., Goodman, T., Creswell, D., Tillisch, K., Mayer, E. A. and Naliboff, B. D. (2011). Impact of mindfulness-based stress reduction training on intrinsic brain connectivity. *NeuroImage* 56, pp. 290-298.

Luders, E., Clark, K., Narr, K. L. and Toga, A. W. (2011). Enhanced brain connectivity in long-term meditation practitioners. *NeuroImage*, 57, pp. 1308-1316.

Mazaheri, A., Nieuwenhuis, I. L. C., van Dijk, H. and Jensen, O. (2009). Prestimulus Alpha and Mu Activity Predicts Failure to Inhibit Motor Responses, *Hum. Brain Mapp.,* 30, pp.1791-1800.

McMahon, D. M. (2006). *Happiness: a history.* Atlantic Monthly Press, (New York, USA).

Neiman, S. (2002). *Evil in Modern Thought.* (Princeton University Press, USA).

Raz, A. and Buhle, J. (2006). Typologies of attentional networks, *Nat. Rev. Neurosci.*, 7, pp. 367-379.

Romei, V., Brodbeck, V., Michel, C., Amedi, A., Pascual-Leone, A. *et al.* (2008). Spontaneous fluctuations in posterior alpha-band EEG activity reflect variability in excitability of human visual areas, *Cereb. Cortex,* 18, pp. 2010-2018.

Seeley, W. W., Menon, V., Schatzberg, A. F., Keller, J., Glover, G. H., Heather Kenna, H., Reiss, A. L., Michael, D. and Greicius M. D. (2007). Dissociable Intrinsic Connectivity Networks for Salience Processing and Executive Control, J. *Neurosci.*, 27(9), pp. 2349-2356.

van den Hurk, P., Giommi, F., Gielen, S. C., Speckens, A. E. M. and Barendregt, H. P. (2010). Greater efficiency in attentional processing related to mindfulness meditation, *Quart. J. Exp. Psychol.*, 63 (6), pp. 1168-1180.

Wise, R. A. (2002). Brain reward circuitry: Insights from unsensed incentives. *Neuron*, 36, pp. 229-240.

4 Health of Mind Captured: Brain Trained to Body Talk

Szabolcs Kéri[*]

Department of Cognitive Science, Budapest University of Technology and Economics; National Institute of Psychiatry and Addictions, Budapest, Hungary
szkeri@cogsci.bme.hu

What Kind of Vat is Designed for the Brain by Plato and *Zhōngyī*?

Mental illnesses, including stress- and trauma-related disorders are nowadays conceptualized as diseases of the brain (Andreasen, 1997; Krishnan and Nestler, 2010; Insel and Landis, 2013). A complex interaction among recent and remote life events, continuously and dynamically changing social, economic, and environmental influences, and genetic traits lead to a disturbed balance of neuronal circuits, which are responsible for learning and memory, attention, emotion regulation, social cognition, and eventually the multifaceted representation of the self. The phenomena described by abnormal psychology or psychopathology are ultimate manifestations of the impaired functioning of small-scale and more widely distributed neuronal populations, which can be detected as neurotransmitter imbalances, fine structural alterations of synapses, altered metabolic pathways, and perturbed gene expression regulatory networks (Andreasen, 1997; Krishnan and Nestler, 2010; Insel and Landis, 2013).

Due to our efforts to deeply understand the interaction among environmental factors, brain circuits, and epigenetic regulatory mechanisms, traditionally separate approaches (e.g., social sciences, neurosciences, and genetics) tend to be bound in a cooperative manner. However, there remains a gap between Western systemization and Eastern holism. Since Gilbert Harman's reinterpretation of Descartes' Evil Demon (Harman, 1973), we have learnt that it is quite problematic to describe how a brain isolated not only from its external environment

* Address for correspondence: Department of Cognitive Science, Budapest University of Technology and Economics, Egry str. 1, Budapest, H1111, Hungary.

(sensory input), but also from neurohormonal and visceral interoceptive signals deriving from the *milieu intérieur* ("a brain in the vat") can produce percepts, memories, knowledge, emotions, intentions, and finally a conscious experience of the self and other intelligent agents.

Traditional Western systematization sharply distinguishes our external environment, body, and brain and looks at their communication and interrelatedness via borders, gates, and regulatory mechanisms. In contrast, in Eastern holism parts are less important; the brain and body are embedded in the environment and the brain is embedded in the body – their separate existence has no meaning at all (Nisbett, 2003).

According to the philosophy of Plato (427-347 BC), the human soul has logical, spiritual, and appetitive spheres housed in different parts of the brain and body; the brain, the cathedral of the rational soul, is strictly separated from lower-level mind-modules by the neck. The view of Aristotle (384-322 BC) is quite different postulating that the soul is not a separate substance from that of the body. In ancient Greek, flesh (Sarx, σάρξ) refers to both human body and human nature. The Aristotelian concept of unity had fundamental consequences regarding later Western philosophy, theology, and the roots of Reformation and Enlightenment (McGrath, 2011).

Well before these intellectual streams in the West, in the era of the Shang Dynasty (14-11 cent. BC), *Zhōngyī* (中医), the Traditional Chinese Medicine delineated a fairly different kind of "vat" for the brain: in this model, brain functions are distributed among the five *zhang*-organs (liver, lung, spleen, heart, and kidney), and therefore brain diseases can be considered as systemic processes distributed in the whole body. In the Hindu Ayurveda (5000 BC), the brain is responsible for perception, movements, and rational thinking, and the mind can control the body. Therefore, changes in mind due to meditation, for example, will result in changes in body functions (Patwardhan *et al.*, 2005).

The assumptions discussed above raise several questions that can be addressed by using the tools of modern neuroscience, psychology, and physiology. Frist, what is the effect of environmental shaping of cognition (e.g., during cognitive therapy or mindfulness training) on brain structure and how is it affected by molecular factors playing an important role in the physiological regulation of body functions? Second, what is the relationship between the supposed changes in brain and the internal environment of the body with a special reference to the human gut microbiota and inflammatory mechanisms (the so-called brain-gut axis)?

These questions are essential to understand the mechanism of psychotherapy, among others, in stress- and trauma-related disorders.

Change the Mind if You Cannot Change the World: Cognitive Behavioral Therapy and Mindfulness-Based Approaches

In the 1960-70s, Aaron Beck discovered a very close relationship between thoughts and emotions (Beck, 1976). Beck's approach is fundamentally rational and Western-style: emotional reactions stem from inferences and causal judgments on memories, contexts, and current stimuli. He identified automatic thoughts which are emotion-filled mental contents appearing unintentionally in the field of consciousness. In anxiety and depression, these thoughts are unrealistically biased towards fears and hopelessness/helplessness due to certain cognitive distortions (e.g., overgeneralization of negative outcomes, polarized black-or-white thinking, and early jumping to a conclusion). During cognitive-behavioral therapy (CBT), patients are trained to use practical psychological techniques to identify, evaluate, and change automatic thoughts, attitudes, and behaviors (Beck, 1976).

However, sometimes changing cognitive biases and attitudes is not sufficient: unacceptable memories of traumas and loss cannot be deleted or reframed, and sometimes "biased" and "distorted" cognitions do reflect the situation in a form of depressive and traumatic realism. Using an Eastern approach, in 1979, Jon Kabat-Zinn established an outpatient clinic using the Mindfulness approach, which is based on the Buddhist tradition of Vipassanā (Kabat-Zinn, 2005). In a meditative framework, patients remember major life events, painful and traumatic memories in non-judgmental and non-elaborative manner. They focus on thoughts, feelings, and emotions from a mental distance of the present by remaining contemplative, open, and accepting. Today, third-wave CBT is often used to treat depression and anxiety by amalgamating the approaches of Beck and Kabat-Zinn (Hollon and Ponniah, 2010).

In Beck's new integrative model of depression (Beck and Bredemeier, 2016), the domains of depressogenic beliefs, negative cognitive appraisals, and automatic thoughts are modulated by current stressful events, but, on the other hand, autonomic and immune responses also appear in the form of "sickness behavior" (mental and physical fatigue, decreased motivation, weakened ability to experience pleasure, and poor appetite). It is a very important advancement because psychological constructs are placed in an internal physiological environment. Beck's new model still skips advances in clinical neurochemistry and neuroanatomy, and the neuronal mechanisms of depression are only tangentially and indirectly included. Therefore, by 2016, Beck found a "vat" for thoughts but the brain is still missing.

How can we conceptualize physiologically determined "sickness behavior" in more details? How is it associated with brain structure and function and can it be modified by CBT (i.e., changes in cognitive biases)? Before directly addressing these questions, it is essential to overview a new aspect of our body "vat": the enormously large and complex population of bacteria living in our gastrointestinal system.

A Special Vat for the Brain: The Human Microbiota – Gut – Brain Axis and the Stress Response

Now we know that approximately 100 trillion bacteria live in our intestinal system, which means 4 million extra genes within the human body. Recently, it has been discovered that a special population of viruses regulates the growth of this bacterial population. On the one hand, the human microbiota shows a remarkable stability but also an inter-individual variability, depending on age, nutritional status, and geographical localization. The majority of the bacterial population belongs to the family of Lachnospiraceae, Ruminococcaceae, and other families in Clostridiales. A smaller, but important portion includes Lactobacillaceae, Enterococcaceae, Streptococcaceae, and Veillonellaceae. There is an increasing amount of evidence that the human microbiota is implicated in various neuropsychiatric illnesses, metabolic disturbances, obesity, cancer, autoimmune processes, and allergy (Lozupone *et al.*, 2012; Zhang *et al.*, 2015; Saad *et al.*, 2016).

The gut microbiota contacts with the "second brain", that is, the entire nervous system comprising at least 100 million neurons. Also, stress responses change the homeostatic balance between host and microbiota: circulating catecholamines and cortisol disrupt the integrity of the epithelial barrier in the gut ("leaky gut"), which results in the translocation of bacteria to the submucosa, eliciting an inflammatory response. Consequently, circulating cytokines produce sickness behavior by penetrating the blood-brain-barrier and modulating neuronal activity in the hypothalamus, amygdala, and hippocampus (Maes *et al.*, 2013; Gur and Bailey, 2016).

A critical question is how one can investigate the pathological activation of the microbiota – gut – brain axis. Researchers must face the challenge of overwhelming richness of available data. Although system biology and bioinformatics provide valuable network models for stress markers and inflammatory mechanisms, it is extremely difficult to select key factors that have master-regulatory properties (i.e., hubs in molecular networks) and to provide clinically feasible targets. By critically reviewing "big data" results, we selected six single candidates and a more complex gene expression panel to follow-up stress responses, microbiota activation, and low-grade inflammation in patients with mood and anxiety disorders (Kéri *et al.*, 2014a, b):

- *16s rRNA:* A key component of the bacterial ribosome. By measuring 16s RNA in the blood plasma, one can detect bacterial translocation and the appearance of bacterial components in the circulation.
- *TLR-4* (Toll-Like Receptor-4): A pattern recognition receptor detecting bacterial lipopolysaccharide (LPS) in leukocytes, peripheral circulation, and glial cells in the brain.
- *IL-6* (Interleukin-6): The most abundant circulating cytokine, which mediates many aspects of sickness behavior in the brain.
- *CRP* (C-reactive protein): An acute phase protein produced by the liver as a part of the stress response and inflammation.
- *FKBP5:* A key regulator of the cortisol receptor. FKBP5 can down-regulate the cortisol receptor representing an important negative feedback factor in stress response and inflammation.
- *NF-κβ:* A master regulator transcription factor activated by cytokines in leukocytes and brain. Activated leukocytes during stress response and inflammation produce multiple kinds of cytokines by the activation of the NF-κβ system.

Restoring the Vat via the Brain: Can Psychotherapy Change the Microbiota-Stress Response Activation?

How can we modify and re-balance the above-described microbiota-stress response system? There are multiple attempts to design clinically useful anti-inflammatory medications and cortisol-antagonists to directly restore low-grade inflammation and stress response. More recently, several authors raised the possibility that beneficial probiotic microbes can ameliorate depression and anxiety (the so-called "psychobiotics") (Dinan *et al.*, 2013). Finally, there is a theoretical possibility to restore microbiota-stress responses by psychotherapies such as Beck's CBT. During CBT, which is essentially a learning process dominated by self-monitoring, attentional tuning, and re-appraisal, there is a complex and dynamic change in brain structure and function, which may affect not only cognition and affective regulation, but also the activation of the autonomic nervous system and the hypothalamic-pituitary axis (HPA) (Franklin *et al.*, 2016). In turn, normalization of the autonomic/HPA activation may decrease bacterial translocation and low-grade peripheral inflammation.

First, we tested this hypothesis in patients with major depressive disorder (MDD) who received CBT for 16 weeks (Kéri *et al.*, 2014a). Microbiota-stress response parameters were measured before and after CBT from peripheral blood samples. As shown in Fig. 1(a), we detected 16s rRNA positivity in 78% of our patients, which indicates increased intestinal permeability and bacterial translocation in the majority of newly diagnosed, non-medicated patients with MDD (n=50). Figure 1(a) also shows a significant reduction of 16s rRNA after CBT: only 56% of the patients remained positive for the bacterial marker. Elevated TLR-4 mRNA expression in peripheral lymphocytes confirmed these findings: before CBT, MDD patients exhibited a marked TLR4 activation, which was reduced following the therapy (Fig. 1(b)). Importantly, this effect was not observed for TLR-2 receptors, which are not sensitive for the detection of Gram-negative bacteria from the intestinal flora.

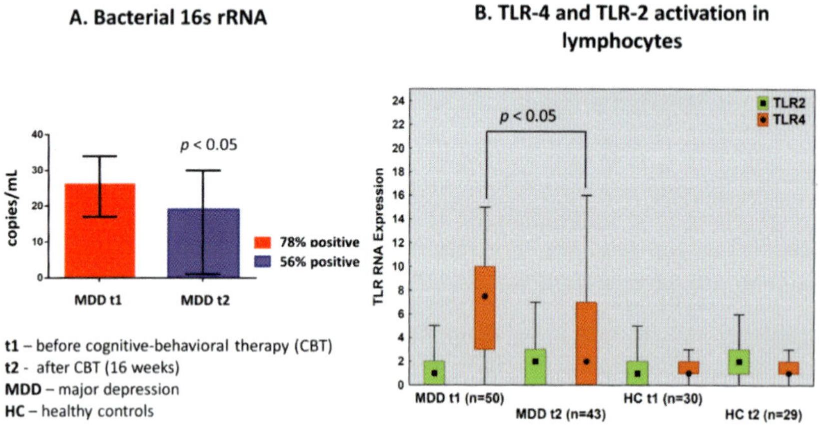

Fig. 1. Bacterial ribosomal RNA and TLR4 receptor activation in depression before and after CBT.

However, TLR-4 is only a single factor, and it is dubious whether lymphocytes really displayed a widespread and definitive immune activation in MDD. To elucidate this issue, we measured NF-κβ activation, as well as the expression of a panel of 10 genes related to growth factor signaling, cytokines, and glial functions *(MBP, EDG2, FZD3, ATXN1, EDNRB, FGFR1, MAG, PMP22, UGT8, ERBB3)* (Kéri *et al.*, 2014b).

In accordance with the findings from the measurement of 16s rRNA and TLR-4, NF-κβ and the 10-item transcriptomics marker scores (BioM10) revealed a definitive lymphocyte activation in non-medicated patients with MDD (Fig. 2). Lower BioM10 scores indicate decreased gene expression in depressed patients, whereas the expression of NF-κβ mRNA was markedly increased. These changes were reversed after CBT: there were significant increases in BioM10 scores and decreases in NF-κβ expression (Fig. 2).

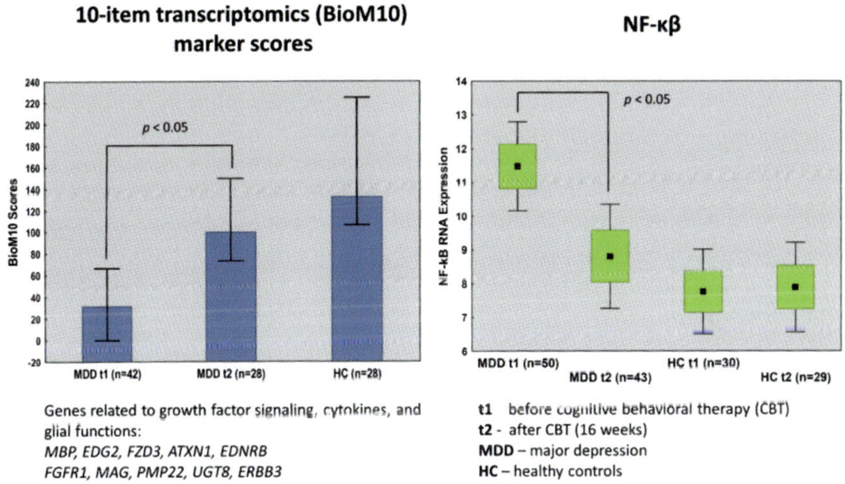

Fig. 2. NF-κβ and other gene expression changes in lymphocytes in depression before and after CBT.

Moreover, changes in TLR-4, BioM10, and NF-κβ expression were associated with clinical improvement during CBT: greater improvement in depression was related to decreased TLR-4 and NF-κβ activation and increased BioM10 scores. Interestingly, it was not the case for two widely used markers of peripheral low-grade inflammation, IL-6 and CRP. These factors did not exhibit convincing and robust alterations, and there was no association between their levels and clinical responses.

Why are these changes important at the biological level and how are they related to each other? Garate *et al.* (2013) developed an animal model of depression, which was based on the phenomenon of increased intestinal permeability. It was found that chronic mild stress increased bacterial LPS in the circulation of rats, colonization of leukocytes in intestinal lymph nodes, activation of the TLR-4 pathway resulting in behavioral desperation. In upstream activation pathways, TLR-4 and its co-receptor, myeloid differentiation protein-2 (MD-2), detect LPS and activate a network including the master-regulator NF-κβ. NF-κβ is a key factor to facilitate the production of cytokines and arachidonic-acid derivates. Garate *et al.* (2013) also showed that stress up-regulates TLR-4 in the frontal cortex of mice resulting in the activation of NF-κβ and pro-inflammatory enzymes (nitric oxide synthase and cyclooxygenase-2). These mechanisms may be related to oxidative and nitrosative cellular damage in the brain. Evidence also indicates that intestinal decontamination with antibiotics prevents stress-induced elevation of LPS binding protein in the circulation and TLR-4 activation in the frontal cortex of experimental animals (Garate *et al.*, 2013).

Changes in the Vat, Changes in the Brain

The studies reported so far indicated how psychological intervention can change low-grade peripheral immune activation, markers of bacterial translocation, and intestinal permeability. However, we have no information how CBT changed brain structure and function in relation to stress response and immune activation. To investigate these possible changes, we selected patients with Posttraumatic Stress Disorder (PTSD) because severe stress exposition is more consistent as compared with MDD in which diffuse and prolonged psychosocial stress can be seen.

PTSD patients report a persistent and disturbing re-experience of traumatic events (e.g., natural disasters, wars, accidents, interpersonal and political violence), avoidance of situations related to the trauma (trauma-related thoughts, feelings, activities; diminished social interest, blunted emotional reactions), and heightened arousal (irritability, sleep disorder, and distractibility). There is evidence that CBT alters brain activation in prefrontal and cingulate areas of PTSD patients, whereas volumetric changes are mainly confined to cingulate regions and the hippocampal formation (Quidé *et al.*, 2012).

How are these changes related to the activation of the stress response system? Beyond the measurement of cortisol levels, FKBP5 (FK506 binding protein) may be a key candidate to understand how the stress axis is perturbed in PTSD. FKBP5 is an intracellular protein binding to the glucocorticoid receptor complex and can decrease cortisol affinity and the nuclear translocation of the receptor. Therefore, a decreased expression of FKBP5 results in receptor overactivity and a heightened sensitivity of the HPA for negative feedback by glucocorticoids. Genetic polymorphisms of the *FKBP5* gene interact with environmental trauma exposure and increase vulnerability for PTSD (Mehta and Binder, 2012).

Taking these findings together, we delineated the following framework of hypotheses (Levy-Gigi *et al.*, 2013):

(i) In PTSD patients without medications and psychological treatment, there is a decreased level of peripheral FKBP5 expression, which results in the overactivity of the HPA.

(ii) It is well known that the hippocampus is one of the most vulnerable brain structures in relation to stress and increased glucocorticoid response in the HPA. Therefore, it is plausible to hypothesize that decreased FKBP5 (hypersensitive HPA) correlates with hippocampal volume loss in PTSD.

(iii) If these mechanisms are valid, CBT may be able to normalize FKBP5 expression and hippocampal volume.

(iv) Finally, we proposed that overactive stress response in PTSD is accompanied by increased intestinal permeability and bacterial translocation.

Figure 3 summarizes the key results. First, similar to MDD (Kéri *et al.*, 2014a), patients with PTSD had increased intestinal permeability as revealed by positivity for bacterial 16s rRNA at t1 (baseline, before CBT). The post-CBT data (t2) were also in accordance with the findings from MDD: we observed a significant decline in 16s rRNA, which suggests that intestinal permeability showed a tendency of normalization during CBT (Levy-Gigi *et al.*, 2013).

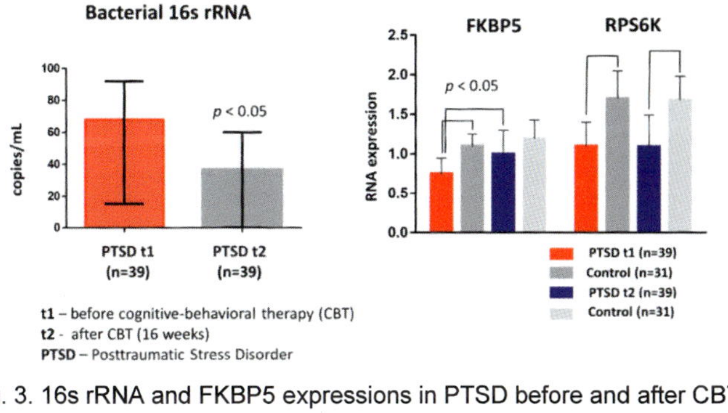

Fig. 3. 16s rRNA and FKBP5 expressions in PTSD before and after CBT.

FKBP5 expression was contrasted with RPS6K expression, a human ribosomal factor previously found to be associated with PTSD (Yehuda *et al.*, 2009). Briefly, FKBP5 appeared to be a state marker, whereas RPS6K remained the same despite CBT. As expected, patients with PTSD were characterized by low FKBP5 before CBT, which was normalized after CBT. RPS6K was lower in patients with PTSD relative to the controls at both before and after CBT.

These findings indicate that in newly diagnosed patients with PTSD (no history of psychotropic medications and psychological treatments), there is a hyperactivity of the HPA as indicated by a decreased expression of FKBP5, a negative regulator of the glucocorticoid receptor. This marker seems to be much robust than plasma cortisol levels. This is consistent with previous results from the literature. For example, Segman *et al.* (2005) found that *FKBP5* gene expression, within a few hours after a traumatic event, correlated with the severity of acute posttraumatic symptoms. Yehuda *et al.* (2009) reported lower *FKBP5* RNA levels in PTSD patients surviving the attack against the World Trade Center. These human studies are consistent with animal models indicating that the *FKBP5* gene is expressed together with glucocorticoid receptors in PTSD-associated brain structures, including the hippocampal formation and the central amygdala (Scharf *et al.*, 2011).

The next question we addressed was related to changes in brain structure during CBT in PTSD (Levy-Gigi *et al.*, 2013). We focused on three key structures implicated in the functional neuroanatomy of PTSD: medial prefrontal cortex, hippocampus, and amygdala. The medial prefrontal cortex is important in affective regulation providing a higher-order input to the amygdala. For example, medial prefrontal-amygdala connections are critical in the extinction of negative fear memories. Hippocampal atrophy is one of the most frequently found and replicated findings in stress- and trauma-related disorders including PTSD. The hippocampus is critical not only in the establishment of episodic memories but also in multisensory integration, and the ventral parts of it are related to the regulation of the HPA and stress response in PTSD (Pitman *et al.*, 2012; Li *et al.*, 2014).

Regarding the morphological correlates of CBT, we reported a simple and circumscribed phenomenon: there was a significantly increased hippocampal volume in PTSD patients after they completed CBT. The orbitofrontal cortex and the amygdala did not show any change. However, as a standalone finding, this is not surprising given the well-known role of the hippocampus in trauma-related disorders. A more interesting aspect of our result is a three-way correlation among changes in hippocampal volume, FKBP5 expression, and PTSD symptoms during CBT. Figure 4 illustrates how these measures are related to each other: greater improvement in PTSD symptoms was associated with more enhanced FKBP5 expression and increased hippocampal volume (Levy-Gigi *et al.*, 2013).

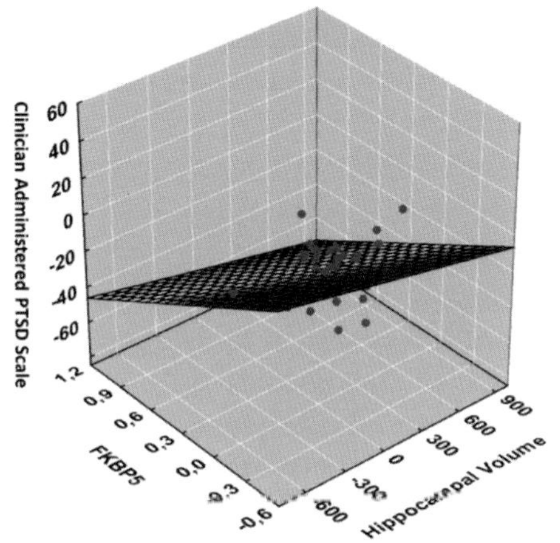

Fig. 4. Correlation among PTSD symptom changes, hippocampal volume, and FKBP5 expression during CBT.

The causal relationship among PTSD symptoms, hippocampal volume, and FKBP5 is not clear. The most likely scenario is that CBT exerts its primary effect on the functional activation of the prefrontal-amygdala-hippocampal network, which will lead to the normalization of the HPA stress system. Changes in FKBP5 expression may be a key molecular component of HPA normalization. Next, after the re-balancing of the HPA, hippocampal atrophy will be ameliorated because the toxic effect of the hyperactive glucocorticoid (HPA) system will be turned down. At the level of the body, down-regulated glucocorticoid activity may explain why we observed a reduced microbiota translocation given that the overactive stress system can induce increased gastrointestinal permeability by disrupting the gut epithelial barrier.

These findings raise several important therapeutic targets that may enhance the effect of CBT. One may hypothesize that drugs affecting FKBP5 may be particularly powerful. Alternative possibilities are food supplementation with probiotics, as well as changes in diet, to restore gut microbiota, or anti-inflammatory agents reducing the harmful consequences of bacterial translocation. In animals, antibiotic intestinal decontamination was also useful and reduced anxiety and depressive symptoms (Garate *et al.*, 2013), but in humans such treatment interventions have inherent limitations.

Basic Brain Train when Life is not Bright

There is no doubt that CBT requires the coordinated action of multiple basic cognitive functions: when patients monitor their inner dialogue, retrieve and re-evaluate personal memories, and focus on the emotional value and outcome of decisions and appraisals, they use attention, executive functions, episodic memory, language, and theory of mind faculties. If basic cognitive functions are impaired, CBT may be less effective. Recently, there is extensive and emerging public interest in various cognitive enhancement and "brain train" methods not only to improve basic cognition in neuropsychiatric illnesses but also to boost normal cognition to achieve better performance in everyday life. There is a remarkable controversy in the interpretation of outcome, usefulness, and generalizability of these publicly available computerized games, and it is less known how they may affect brain structure and function (Owen *et al.*, 2010).

Kühn *et al.* (2014) obtained brain images from a group of individuals who were trained on a popular platformer game (Super Mario) for 2 months. As compared to control individuals, trained subjects showed significant gray matter increases in the right hippocampus, dorsolateral prefrontal cortex, and bilateral cerebellum. The game involves spatial navigation and shifting allocentric and egocentric strategies during the navigation of an animated character, and, hence, it is not surprising that right hippocampal changes correlated with these spatial navigation measures.

However, the Kühn *et al.* (2014) study had an interesting affective aspect: the desire for video gaming correlated with gray matter changes. Motivation and desire are sensitively related to mood states, and adverse life events causing even subclinical depressive and anxiety experiences may disrupt pleasure-seeking behavior. It is needless to state that adverse life events have a significant impact on the "vat" of the brain, that is, our internal physiological environment. This is best characterized by the activation of lymphocytes as indicated by elevated NF-κβ expression.

The question is how structural changes in the brain during cognitive training are related to adverse life events and consequent pro-inflammatory responses.

We investigated 56 healthy individuals who participated in two-month Super Mario training (30 min/day) (Szabó *et al.*, 2014). As expected, there was a significant expansion of the right hippocampal formation, but it was modulated by both psychosocial and inflammatory measures. Individuals who experienced more negative life events during the past year exhibited less pronounced hippocampal volume expansion. It seems that increased NF-κβ mediated this effect, and common measures of peripheral low-grade inflammation (IL-6 and CRP) were not dominantly related to gray matter changes (Fig. 5.).

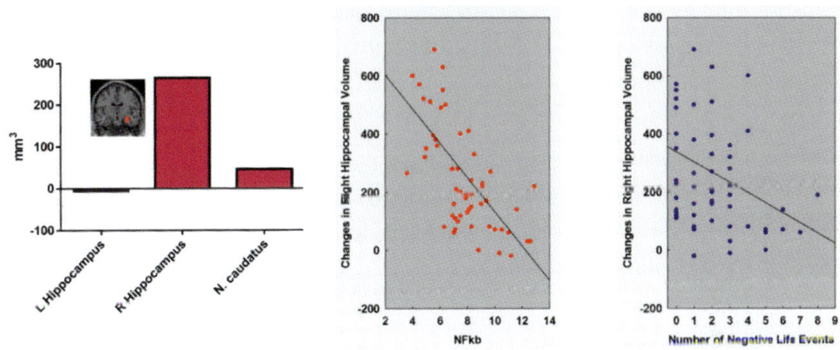

Fig. 5. Changes in right hippocampal volume (mm^3) during cognitive training and its relationship with adverse negative life events and NF-κβ expression.

It is worthy to note that volume changes during training were not generalized. As shown in Fig. 5, we observed no significant changes in the volume of the caudate nucleus despite the fact that this brain structure is implicated not only in motor planning and control but also some aspects of spatial navigation (West *et al.*, 2015). A possible explanation is that our platformer game required allocentric-egocentric spatial navigation strategies that are less habitual and requires the establishment of an actively monitored internal cognitive map of the environment. The hippocampus is especially critical for such type of cognition whereas the caudate nucleus may be responsible for more habitual, less flexible but stable reward-guided learning (West *et al.*, 2015).

Correlations among peripheral markers, brain structure, and psychological functions must always be treated with caution because we have no direct evidence on pro-inflammatory changes in the brain. Nevertheless, NF-κβ participates in the homeostatic regulation of neurons in the hippocampal formation, which is a sensitive brain structure for systemic inflammation. Koo *et al.* (2010) demonstrated that stress can activate NF-κβ and consequently impair cell division and plasticity in the hippocampus. NF-κβ is a molecular bridge between depression and chronic stress by affecting neurogenesis, neuronal growth, and learning and memory (Crampton and O'Keeffe, 2013). These animal studies provide further explanation why the negative relationship between hippocampal enlargement and stressful life events was mediated by NF-κβ in our study.

Beyond our results, multiple lines of evidence from human studies support the role of NF-κβ in stress response and neuronal plasticity. There are various psychosocial stressors that activate NF-κβ and pro-inflammatory response: social rejection, childhood abuse, interpersonal conflict with spouses and friends, providing care for individuals with severe illness, low socioeconomic status, and loneliness (Chen and Miller, 2013). It has also been demonstrated that stressful life events have a detrimental effect on human brain structure even when there are no marked psychological and behavioral symptoms (Cohen *et al.*, 2006). Here, we showed that impaired brain plasticity under psychosocial stress is mediated by pro-inflammatory mechanisms, which is consistent with our data from patients with MDD and PTSD (Levy-Gigi *et al.*, 2013; Kéri *et al.*, 2014a, b).

We also showed that CBT is effective in the reduction of the pro-inflammatory response (Kéri *et al.*, 2014a, b). This story has an Eastern side, too. A group of individuals under a serious psychosocial stress (dementia caregivers) received either Kirtan Kriya Meditation or relaxing music. After two months, genome-wide transcriptional profiles and promoter-based bioinformatics analyses revealed that gene expression alterations were driven by reduced activity of the pro-inflammatory NF-κβ (Black *et al.*, 2013). Altogether, there were 68 genes that were differentially expressed after meditation.

What have We Learnt about the Brain in its Vat?

The series of studies summarized above might provide some new insight on the relationship among environment, brain, and body. Herein, the world — the external environment — produces information flow resulting in learning and modification of external or internal behavior. In our studies, these learning processes included a computer game requiring spatial navigation and CBT requiring the internal monitoring of thoughts and emotions and their cognitive reappraisal. Both learning processes were associated with structural changes in the hippocampal formation, which is not surprising given that this highly plastic structure participates in learning, memory, spatial cognition, and emotion regulation.

However, the changes were not confined to the brain: we observed significant alterations in the "vat of the brain", that is, our internal physiological environment. First, one of the key molecular elements of the HPA-immune interactions – FKBP5 – was enhanced by CBT down-regulating the cortisol receptor in lymphocytes. Second, CBT also tampered down innate immune activation (TLR-4), pro-inflammatory transcriptional responses (NF-κβ), and bacterial translocation in the gut. The most likely cascade of events includes an altered activity of key brain regions during CBT (e.g., prefrontal and cingulate cortex, amygdala, and hippocampus) resulting in the down-regulation of the HPA stress system. Finally, the normalization of the HPA system may lead to immune changes and decreased bacterial translocation in the gut (restoration of the "leaky gut").

Beyond the possibility that these results might provide new therapeutic targets that may boost the effectiveness of CBT in PTSD and MDD (e.g., drugs modulating FKBP5, or probiotics regulating microbiota), the findings demonstrate that, by the integration of psychology, neuroscience, and physiology, the gap between Eastern holism and Western systemization can be bridged. In everyday circumstances, the environment, the brain, and the organs of the body form a unique system in which the information flow is continuous and multidirectional. An intensive and fruitful conversation between Eastern and Western traditions will, therefore, provide new insights and solutions regarding complex disorders such as PTSD and MDD.

References

Andreasen, N. C. (1997). Linking mind and brain in the study of mental illnesses: a project for a scientific psychopathology, *Science*, 275, pp. 1586-1593.

Beck, A. T. (1976). *Cognitive Therapy and the Emotional Disorders,* (International University Press, USA).

Beck, A. T. and Bredemeier, K. (2016). A unified model of depression: Integrating clinical, cognitive, biological, and evolutionary perspectives. *Clin. Psychol. Sci.*, Advance online publication, doi:10.1177/2167702616628523.

Black, D. S., Cole, S. W., Irwin, M. R., Breen, E., St Cyr, N. M., Nazarian, N., Khalsa, D. S. and Lavretsky, H. (2013). Yogic meditation reverses NF-κB and IRF-related

transcriptome dynamics in leukocytes of family dementia caregivers in a randomized controlled trial, *Psychoneuroendocrinology,* 38, pp. 348-355.
Cohen, R. A., Grieve, S., Hot, K. F., Paul, R. H., Swee, L., Tate, D., Gunstad, J., Stroud, L., McCaffery, J., Hitsman, B., Niaura, R., Clark, C. R., McFarlane, A., Bryant, R., Gordon, E. and Williams, L. M. (2006). Early life stress and morphometry of the adult anterior cingulate cortex and caudate nuclei, *Biol. Psychiatry,* 59, pp. 975-982.
Crampton, S. J. and O'Keeffe, G. W. (2013). NF-κB: emerging roles in hippocampal development and function, *Int. J. Biochem. Cell Biol.,* 45, 1821-1824.
Dinan, T. G., Stanton, C. and Cryan, J. F. (2013). Psychobiotics: a novel class of psychotropic, *Biol. Psychiatry*, 74, pp. 720-726.
Franklin, G., Carson, A. J. and Welch, K. A. (2016). Cognitive behavioural therapy for depression: systematic review of imaging studies, *Acta Neuropsychiatr.,* 28, pp. 61-74.
Garate, I., Garcia-Bueno, B., Madrigal, J. L., Caso, J. R., Alou, L., Gomez-Lus, M. L., Micó, J. A. and Leza, J. C. (2013). Stress-induced neuroinflammation: role of the Toll-like receptor-4 pathway, *Biol. Psychiatry,* 73, pp. 32-43.
Gur, T. L. and Bailey, M. T. (2016). Effects of stress on commensal microbes and immune system activity, *Adv. Exp. Med. Biol.,* 874, pp. 289-300.
Harman, G. (1973). *Thought*, Princeton University Press.
Hollon, S. D. and Ponniah, K. (2010). A review of empirically supported psychological therapies for mood disorders in adults. *Depress. Anxiety*, 27, pp. 891-932.
Insel, T. R. and Landis, S. C. (2013). Twenty-five years of progress: the view from NIMH and NINDS, *Neuron*, 80, pp. 561-567.
Kabat-Zinn, J. (2005). Full Catastrophe Living: Using the Wisdom of Your Body and Mind to Face Stress, Pain and Illness, 15th Anniversary Ed., Random House.
Kéri, S., Szabó, C. and Kelemen, O. (2014a). Expression of Toll-Like Receptors in peripheral blood mononuclear cells and response to cognitive-behavioral therapy in major depressive disorder, *Brain Behav. Immun.*, 40, pp. 235-243.
Kéri, S., Szabó, C. and Kelemen, O. (2014b). Blood biomarkers of depression track clinical changes during cognitive-behavioral therapy, *J. Affect. Disord.*, 164, pp. 118-122.
Koo, J. W., Russo, S. J., Ferguson, D., Nestler, E. J. and Duman, R. S. (2010). Nuclear factor-kappaB is a critical mediator of stress-impaired neurogenesis and depressive behavior, *Proc. Natl. Acad. Sci. USA,* 107, pp. 2669-2674.
Krishnan, V. and Nestler, E. J. (2010). Linking molecules to mood: new insight into the biology of depression, *Am. J. Psychiatry*, 167, pp. 1305-1320.
Kühn, S., Gleich, T., Lorenz, R. C., Lindenberger, U. and Gallinat, J. (2014). Playing Super Mario induces structural brain plasticity: gray matter changes resulting from training with a commercial video game, *Mol. Psychiatry,* 19, pp. 265-271.
Levy-Gigi, E., Szabó, C., Kelemen, O. and Kéri, S. (2013). Association among clinical response, hippocampal volume, and FKBP5 gene expression in individuals with posttraumatic stress disorder receiving cognitive behavioral therapy, *Biol Psychiatry,* 74, pp. 793-800.
Li, L., Wu, M., Liao, Y., Ouyang, L., Du, M., Lei, D., Chen, L., Yao, L., Huang, X. and Gong, Q. (2014). Grey matter reduction associated with posttraumatic stress disorder and traumatic stress, *Neurosci. Biobehav. Rev.*, 43, pp. 163-172.
Lozupone, C. A., Stombaugh, J. I., Gordon, J. I., Jansson, J. K. and Knight, R. (2012). Diversity, stability and resilience of the human gut microbiota, *Nature,* 489, pp. 220-230.
McGrath, A. E. (2011). *Christian Theology. An Introduction*, 5th ed., Wiley-Blackwell.
Mehta, D. and Binder, E. B. (2012). Gene × environment vulnerability factors for PTSD: the HPA-axis, *Neuropharmacology,* 62, pp. 654-662.
Nisbett, R. (2003). *The Geography of Thought*, The Free Press.

Owen, A. M., Hampshire, A., Grahn, J. A., Stenton, R., Dajani, S., Burns, A. S., Howard, R. J. and Ballard, C. G. (2010). Putting brain training to the test, *Nature,* 465, pp. 775-778.

Patwardhan, B., Dnyaneshwar Warude, D., Pushpangadan, P. and Bhatt, N. (2005). Ayurveda and Traditional Chinese Medicine: a comparative overview, *Evid. Based Complement. Alternat. Med.*, 2, pp. 465-473.

Pitman, R. K., Rasmusson, A. M., Koenen, K. C., Shin, L. M., Orr, S. P., Gilbertson, M. W., Milad, M. R. and Liberzon, I. (2012). Biological studies of post-traumatic stress disorder, *Nat. Rev. Neurosci.,* 13, pp. 769-787.

Quidé, Y., Witteveen, A. B., El-Hage, W., Veltman, D. J. and Olff, M. (2012). Differences between effects of psychological versus pharmacological treatments on functional and morphological brain alterations in anxiety disorders and major depressive disorder: a systematic review, *Neurosci. Biobehav. Rev.*, 36, 626-644.

Saad, M. J., Santos, A. and Prada, P. O. (2016). Linking gut microbiota and inflammation to obesity and insulin resistance. *Physiology (Bethesda),* 31, pp. 283-293.

Scharf, S. H., Liebl, C., Binder, E. B., Schmidt, M. V. and Müller, M. B. (2011). Expression and regulation of the Fkbp5 gene in the adult mouse brain, *PLoS One*, 6, e16883.

Segman, R. H., Shefi, N., Goltser-Dubner, T., Friedman, N., Kaminski, N. and Shalev, A. Y. (2005). Peripheral blood mononuclear cell gene expression profiles identify emergent post-raumatic stress disorder among trauma survivors, *Mol. Psychiatry*, 10, pp. 425.

Szabó, C., Kelemen, O. and Kéri, S. (2014). Low-grade inflammation disrupts structural plasticity in the human brain, *Neuroscience,* 275, pp. 81-88.

West, G. L., Drisdelle, B. L., Konishi, K., Jackson, J., Jolicoeur, P. and Bohbot, V. D. (2015). Habitual action video game playing is associated with caudate nucleus-dependent navigational strategies, *Proc. Biol. Sci.,* 282, 20142952.

Yehuda, R., Cai, G., Golier, J. A., Sarapas, C., Galea, S., Ising, M. *et al.* (2009). Gene expression patterns associated with posttraumatic stress disorder following exposure to the World Trade Center attacks, *Biol. Psychiatry*, 66, pp. 708-711.

Zhang, Y. J., Li, S., Gan, R. Y., Zhou, T., Xu, D. P. and Li, H. B. (2015). Impacts of gut bacteria on human health and diseases. *Int. J. Mol. Sci.,* 16, pp. 7403-7510.

5 Analytic versus Holistic? An Analysis of Some Proposals for Cognitive East-West Differences

Csaba Pléh

Department of Cognitive Science
Central European University, Budapest
vispleh@ceu.edu

I shall start off from three approaches to the thought/culture relations. One is unconstrained universalism, the other is the assumption of qualitative differences between types of thoughts that would by some interpretations correspond to patterns of culture and finally, the third approach allows a multiplicity of styles of thought that can be combined in flexible ways.

As empirical illustration of these assumptions I shall first characterize some proposals for postulating a perceptual, cultural and contextual analyticity/holism strategy difference that is many times related to assume East/West cultural differences. Then I shall move on to what the issue of linguistic relativity taught us about dangers of relating typological differences, and even differences in processing regarding assumed overall geographic/cultural differences. Considering language, the entire issue of East-West differences as related to processing differences becomes rather clumsy, since language typological differences do not in a clear sense correspond to cultural East-West differences in Eurasian or elsewhere.

I shall argue on the basis of our own researches and from studies of other groups for a constrained relativity view, and for a proposal that the processing differences are not absolute, and they are unrelated to clear (or mushy) geographic distinctions.

Perception, Cognition and Sensitivity to Context

The universalistic assumption regarding thought pattern claims is that we are in fact universally rational beings, and our processes of thinking and the resulting world of internal representations are not affected by our social, cultural and emotional contexts. The opposite claim is that the human mind is entirely flexible, being under the control of the cultural environment, and even our most basic competences such as color vision would depend, for example, on the availability of color terms, thus in a way on culture. The mind and brain would be entirely formed under the impact of culture (Cole and Scribner, 1974 presented a by now classical version of these claims).

Framed in another terminology, this relates to the issue whether the human mind has a thoroughly modular organization that is unaffected by culture (Sperber, 1994, 2000), or, according to the opposite radical view, modular organization of the human mind and brain is entirely influenced in a top down manner by the cultural context, and our supposedly primary modules would be modified under the influence of culture. According to a view full of compromises, there are certainly primary or elementary networks, or if you like, modules in the human nervous system that are not easily influenced by cultural context. However, many of the important human achievements are influenced by culture on the level where the outputs of this elementary processing are used for conscious and self-related integration (Hirschfeld, 1994). Cultural patterns do have an influence but not in an entirely thorough top down manner. As Sperber and Hirschfeld (2004) pointed out, many varieties of culture are in fact based on using our modules in an extended manner. The "proper function" is extended to an "actual function". Thus, for example, the primary face recognition mechanisms and the baby face preferences are overused by the Hollywood stylists. Put in another way of argumentation, Norenzayan and Heine (2005) showed that in fact there are different layers of universality. Sometimes, a competence may exist universally, but not being used in each culture, sometimes it is used but for different functions in different cultural contexts, and sometimes it has the same prevalence in different cultures.

There is a much discussed line of research which tries to relate these ideas to the differences between so-called Eastern and Western approaches to different perceptual and cognitive tasks. These are the studies done mainly by Richard Nisbett and his followers which start from the idea that there is an opposition between a supposed Eastern and Western mind, summarized in Table 1.

Table 1. The juxtaposition of Western and Eastern mind proposed by Nisbett (2003, Nisbett and Matsuda, 2003).

Eastern mind	**Western mind**
Relation oriented	Item oriented
Prototype oriented	Feature oriented
Attention to whole	Attention to elements
Social life less individual	Extremely individualized

Nisbett (2003) proposed this series of oppositions as a sort of diverging world views. Easterners are assumed to be more context sensitive, including social contexts, and thereby socially more authority oriented, while Westerners pay more attention to items and categories, therefore they are less sensitive to contexts, including social contexts, and therefore they are cognitively more analytic and socially more individualistic. The opposition also entails some crucial cognitive consequences. In Nisbett's presentation, the causal chain assumed to be that culture basically has an impact on the primary cognitive processes by directing our attention. So attention is directed more to contexts and relations in Easterners, and it is more directed to elements and ignores context. Let me show a few examples from the studies of the group of Nisbett. In most of the studies, subjects are presented with varying stimulus displays, either of a perceptual or of a semantic/logical kind, where the contrast is based on belongingness or inference relying on an item based rule, or on prototype based similarity or natural veracity. One example from Norenzayan *et al.* (2002) is shown in Fig. 1, where the two arrangements differ in what unifies the items. The task is to place the test item in one of the groups.

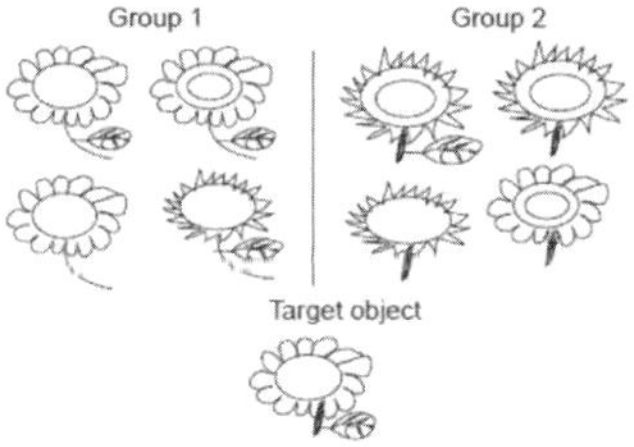

Fig. 1. A task of belongingness based on overall prototype similarity (Group 1), or item similarity (Group 2) (Norenzayan *et al.*, 2002).

Subjects are presented with a target object (in this case, a flower), and they have to decide whether the target belongs to Group 1 or Group 2. The results show that 'white Americans' prefer in 68 % the item based solution, while Asians in 60 % the prototype similarity solution. A sort of larger culture/family culture interaction is shown by the fact that Asian Americans show a 55/45 % distribution, slightly preferring the prototype based solution.

A similar study by the group of Nisbett (Nisbett and Masuda, 2003) had subjects watch short videos of complex visual scenes such as an aquarium. In a free recall situation, Americans started their report of what they saw with the relatively big sized stimuli. Japanese subjects started more with details, and they mentioned twice as frequently the relations between objects and the background as Americans did. In recognition tests where the target object and the background were manipulated, Japanese subjects made 60 % recognition errors based on context dependency.

Similar studies also showed eye movement differences. 'White Americans' showed more fixations to target objects, while Japanese subjects fixated more on the background (Chua *et al.*, 2005).

Nisbett based his generalizing claims on a good dozen of perceptual and cognitive studies. The Eastern approach to perceptual and cognitive tasks is more context oriented, and it is even more field dependent. This is related to the fact that social considerations direct attention to relations in East Asian people and cultures. In the Western orientation, there is a more individualistic social orientation that is directing our attention and perception more towards details.

As the Nisbett group summarized their attitude: "It is common to consider such factors in high-level cognition, but because such factors can influence the allocation of attention, they influence lower level cognition as well. Our hypothesis is that differential attention to context and object are stressed through socialization practices, as demonstrated in studies on childrearing practices by East Asians and Americans. The childrearing practices are, in turn, influenced by societal differences. East Asians live in relatively complex social networks with prescribed role relations. Attention to context is, therefore, important for effective functioning. In contrast, Westerners live in less constraining social worlds that stress independence and allow them to pay less attention to context" (Chua *et al.*, 2005, p. 12633).

The Nisbett style claims regarding East-West differences can be criticized from several perspectives.

1. *Cultural variety.* One limitation of the operationalization of his attitude should be constantly emphasized. In most of the empirical studies, Eastern mind and Eastern perception is studied in East Asian subjects, mostly Chinese and Japanese people. This limitation is a social and geographical oversimplification of the East-West dimension, and East-West itself as an oversimplification of cultural variety. It is of course too easy to characterize Western and Eastern as being two homogeneous populations. Actually Nisbett was trying to soften his position. His group made some studies in Eastern Europe, in the Balkan area (Varnum *et al.*, 2008) basically showing that people from the Balkan area are showing a more versatile or more mixed attitude, compared to West Europeans, showing more cognitive holism, in line with their assumed more social interdependency.
2. The issue of *variation within cultures.* In the much cited holistic versus analytic perceptual strategies opposition one is reminded

that similar ideas have been proposed in the relationships between personality and perception for quite a long time. In the framework of the organismic-physiognomic perceptual theory proposed by Werner and Wapner (1949) and Witkin *et al.* (1972), even some of the tasks are similar to the ones applied by the Nisbett group, like the Rod and Frame test. Thus, the whole idea that there are more contextual and less contextual people in the treatment of their experiences is not entirely tied to culture, but is a complex function, which is partly dependent on culture, partly on personality, and partly on gender (Kimchi *et al.*, 2009).

3. The social claims underlying their assumed cultural differences are also non digital. They are not all or none style, and they are characteristic of both Eastern and Western social integration. Chan and Yan (2007, p. 398) list these assumed features regarding Eastern style. (1) The presence of 'Eastern' dialecticism; (2) The preference to reach a compromise instead of creating a confrontation; (3) The preference to focus on divergent aspects of *apparently* contradictory statements in order to avoid confrontation; and, (4) The preference to willingly interpret statements in order to dissolve the apparent.

These features do characterize Western rhetorical strategies many times as well. Contradictions are tolerated sometimes by Westerners as well. "The so-called 'Eastern' style of thinking can also be found in the thinking patterns of Westerners, the differences identified by Nisbett are often differences in degree rather than in kind." (Ibid, p 398). Differences in attitude towards rival claims can also be explained socially. "Chinese people might be more in favor of striking a compromise in order to maintain harmonious relations. Choosing the middle way or following the mean is a thinking strategy that is adaptive to a social environment which treasures harmony. From a logical point of view, this thinking style, as we have argued, is no less logical than that of the American subjects in Nisbett's experiment" (Ibid, p. 400).

Analytic and Holistic in Language Processing

I move on to studies of differences in language and its relationship to thought. Regarding the relationship between perception, thought and language, there is a long tradition from the early 19th century and so on from Wilhelm von Humboldt (1836) and then on the American scene, from the work of Whorf (1939, 1941) who has sort of rejuvenated these ideas in the 1930's. The basic idea was that language determines thought and this is shown in the fact of grammatical and lexical effects on different aspects of human cognition.

The original ideas proposed by Humboldt and Whorf were rather abstract, with certain circularity because they were not proposing clear behavioral claims. As Lenneberg (1953, p. 463) put this issue in a trend setting paper "a demonstration that certain languages differ from each other suggests but does not prove that the speakers of these languages differ from each other as a group in their psychological potentialities. To prove this, it would be necessary to show first that certain aspects of language have a direct influence on or connection with a given psychological mechanism or at least those speakers of different languages differ along certain psychological parameters". From the mid-20th century on, this very idea whether language has a relevant influence on our perception and cognition, has been articulated more using exact behavioral measures. For a historical analysis of the entire idea of the Whorf hypothesis, Kay and Kempton (1984) gives a good analysis, while Miller and MacNeill (1968) survey the early behavioral interpretations. The reader by Fuchs and Robert (1999) presents later, more grammar related developments.

There were two research efforts in interpreting the Whorf claim in an operationalized behavioral manner. Some studies looked for lexical influences, like the impact of color terms on color memory (for a considerate analysis of many dozen studies see (Rosch, 1975) and a review by Lucy and Shweder (1979)), while others were looking for impacts of grammatical organization on thought, like the impact of grammatical coding of the shape of objects in verbal conjugation on the shape based classifications (Carroll and Casagrande, 1958). Different research outlooks have taken shape, and partly also followed each other. First in the 1950's, many people were claiming that there are large differences due to language resulting in an overall relativity. Language sort of determines the way we perceive the world. Then in the 60's under the influence of the universalistic trend initiated by Chomsky (1965, 1966, 1986, 1988), relativity was replaced by universalistic ideas accompanied by a modularity claim (Fodor, 1983). For this view, we have to look for biologically based universal models of cognition. At the same time, regarding the language/perception/thought interface, their independence as claimed by the new cognitive trends. Language and perception are two different domains in this vision, thus one can talk of a 'BIG MODULARITY' between them, while the internal components of the language system entail a 'SMALL MODULARITY', syntax, phonology, semantic working independently on their own.

This was followed later by more organized typological studies looking for typological effects of language types on cognition in specified areas, like the program of Levinson (1996) on spatial cognition and space coding in languages.

In the entire process of trying to relate thinking and language, the different poles of the relationships are being given rival interpretations.

1. *What is thinking?* Is it a comprehensive world view, as implied by Whorf, or a system of representations, as taken by Fodor (2008) in his Language of Thought vision in the strict sense, or is it rather problem solving?
2. *Language* can also have several interpretations here. Are we talking of the grammatical system, or its actual use, i.e. speech, and especially inner speech, and regarding the use of language, do we consider the rhetoric and pragmatic aspects as well, or merely lexical and grammatical aspects?
3. *The influence* is also rather variedly interpreted. It may suggest that language is a necessary precondition of thought, or a usual instrument, or a tool that merely shapes our thought processes. When it is needed we use it, otherwise we do overcome its influence. According to some strong interpretations, language is the prison of thought, according to others, it is the midwife.

Table 2 summarizes the empirical translations of the language /thought interface into issues of the impact of differences between languages over a half century. In the following I shall mainly talk about the last two lines, since that is where my researches are.

Table 2. Some major empirical translations of the relativity/universalism claims. After Pléh (2000).

Typical research issues	**Actual research**
Circularities in the Whorfian argumentation: language causes mental differences which are seen in language	Lenneberg (1953)
Empirical operationalization *Lexicon*: codability effects *Grammar*: grammatical structure and category learning	Brown and Lenneberg (1954), Lantz and Stefflre (1964), Carroll and Casagrande (1958)
Softened relativism: language fosters when used	Miller and MacNeill (1968)

Table 2. (*Continued*)

Typical research issues	Actual research
Cross linguistic differences in language processing: language-language relativism	Slobin and Bever (1982), Bates and MacWhinney (1989), Gergely and Pléh (1994)
Orientational relativism: languages direct the attention and orientation	Levinson (1996) Li and Gleitman (2002) Ivády, Felhősi & Pléh, Cs. (2008)

From the 1980's on, both in linguistic circles and within psychology itself, instead of showing cognitive differences in cognition by speakers of randomly selected languages, more intricate typological ideas have come up.

I am going to show some data on simple sentence interpretation supporting a constrained relativity proposal. Regarding the impact of structural language types on sentence processing basically two rival approaches developed over two decades that have studied cross linguistic differences both in acquisition and in processing. One of them is holistic, and the other is analytic, to suggest a superficial (and mistaken) similarity with the Eastern-Western thought differences proposed by Nisbett (2003).

1. The holistic approach of Slobin and Bever

On the basis of their empirical studies Slobin and Bever (1982) proposed that in sentence understanding a holistic form based expectation is constructed, and this holistic (canonic) sentence frame image is mapped into the actual perceptual situation, the state of affairs in the real world. The process of understanding in this approach is basically a template matching procedure, and the measure of understanding is a goodness of fit measure.

While each language is assumed to have a set of these basic forms, the linguistic foundation of these forms is different in typologically different languages. In morphologically impoverished languages such as English they are based on word order. In English NVN corresponds to Agent Action Object, resulting in difficulties of interpreting passive sentences (Menn, 2000), while in highly case marking languages such as Turkish the canonic forms are based entirely on noun endings. The task of the child is to create these canonical forms, and to map these holistic forms to the already established canonic situational representations. Cross-linguistic differences are mainly related to the differences in what canonic forms are represented by the speakers. As Bever (2013) summarized this approach, canonic forms are needed because they are a good compromise between rule based top down and inductive-statistically based bottom up processes of grammatical pattern formation, thereby providing for ease of acquisition and speed of processing.

2. *The analytic competition model of Bates and MacWhinney*

The alternative *competition model* (MacWhinney *et al.*, 1985, MacWhinney, 1989, MacWhinney and Bates, 1989, Pléh, 1989) claims that understanding depends in an analytic manner on the combination of possible individual cues. The process of understanding rather than being an issue of template matching and goodness of fit, is assumed to be an issue of some weighted sum of probabilistic mappings. There are competitions in this model in two respects: there is a competition for cues for functions, and a competition among the different noun phrases within each sentence. In studying these competitions between the different possible cues to code grammatical relations, grammatical features like word order, case marking, and cognitive features like animacy for example, were manipulated in sentence interpretation studies on children and adults. They observed that speakers in some languages rely more on one cue (order), while in others more on one another (case marking), but these differences are always statistical in nature. Some of them are very reliable, like case marking in Hungarian, but they are never full proof. There is another type of competition in understanding individual sentences. In each sentence the nouns compete for the different grammatical roles (Agent, Object, Instrument), and the winners are those for which the probability of the given cue/function mapping is higher.

Table 3 shows some languages studied within this framework regarding their mostly used cues. Hundreds of children and adults interpreted hundreds of sentences or sentoids (*The pencil chases the boy*) to arrive to this generalization.

Table 3: The dominant sentence interpretation cues in different ages in different languages (MacWhinney and Bates, 1989).

Language	Child	Adult
Turkish	Case > Order	Case > Anim > Order
Hungarian	Anim > Case> Order	Case > Order
Warlpiri	Anim > Case> Order	Case > Anim > Order
Serbian	Anim > Case> Order	Case> Agr > Anim > Order
Dutch	Order > Case > Anim	Case > Order > Anim
French	Order > Anim	Agr > Anim > Order
English	Order > Anim > Agr	Order > Anim > Agr

In Table 3 the upper part starts from languages that rely mainly or exclusively on Case marking, and at the bottom languages that only rely on Word Order. In this regard, one could also interpret these differences by saying that Hungarian is more analytic, while English, for example, is more holistic.

There are further differences even among languages that use case marking to code grammatical relations on noun phrases. MacWhinney *et al.* (1985), and Pléh (1989, 1990) highlighted interesting temporal developmental differences. In Turkish, due to its clear case marking (the accusative is coded by vowels), children become proficient in agent assignment ("who-did-what to-whom") by 2 years of age. Hungarian children also attend a language that uses case marking, but in this language this feature is perceptually less transparent. Accusatives are coded by the *–t* stop consonant that results sometimes in difficult consonant clusters like *tigris-t* 'tigerAcc'. Thus, Hungarian children are tuned to the use of exclusive case marking around 3½ years of age. However, English-speaking children stabilize the order-based strategy around the age of 5.

If we take Hungarian and Warlpiri, young children first use the cognitively based animacy feature, and later they unlearn its use. We know from infancy research that children around eight-ten months already differentiate between animate and inanimate objects. Animates are those which have random changes in their pattern of movements, and inanimates are the ones which have an inertia–based pattern of movement. Since they have this cognitive template of animacy, children in all languages try to start using animacy to break the code in the language. In Hungarian, like in Warlpiri, animacy is important in 2 and a half year olds, but it soon loses its importance. Parallel to the decrease of the role of animacy, case marking increases its importance. As the importance of case marking increases in the mind of children, animacy loses its importance. In the language structure Hungarian, like in most Uralic languages, there are no grammatical animacy effects, like gender agreement, neither do we have lexical animacy. *Skin* and *leather* are the same word in Hungarian, *bőr*. Thus, in Hungarian and in Warlpiri, a cognitively available important resource, animacy loses its importance as the strategy of the children becomes tuned to the most reliable cues to function in the given language. Building up the process of understanding is a rather flexible project.

Comparing these two languages also shows clearly that the language related analytic/holistic processing style issue is unrelated to these cognitively much-emphasized East-West difference. Warlpiri is an Australian Aboriginal language, both geographically and historically unrelated to Hungarian, while Hungarian and Warlpiri speakers are the most similar in sentence processing. So it is not an East-West issue but a perceptual accommodation to the dominant feature of a given language.

Localistic Decisions in Hungarian

Gergely (1991) and Gergely and Pléh (1994) observed the reliance on local factors in actual acoustic sentence listening tasks in Hungarian. Subjects listened to short tests where four syllable morphologically simple (*levendula* 'lavender') and complex (*csókjaidtól* 'kissPossPlurYourFrom') words appeared. During listening, subjects had to indicate the presence of short irrelevant clicks that appeared over different positions. Gergely and Pléh found that RTs for the clicks were slower over grammatical morphemes. This implies that the local computation of grammatical information goes on in an online manner in Hungarian, an agglutinative language with complex word forms. An actual word may have 3-4 grammatical relations coded each by a separate morpheme. Similar effects were also reported by the group of Niemi (Niemi *et al.*, 1994) for Finnish that is also a highly agglutinative language.

Due to the local processing efforts; morphologically complex words would require more resources from the working memory system. Németh *et al.* (2011) analyzed this possibility by testing the recall of morphologically complex and simplex words in Hungarian, while controlling for length, frequency, concreteness, and phonological composition. They found that fewer words were recalled if they included case marking suffixes, and derivations showed an in between position, as presented in Fig. 2.

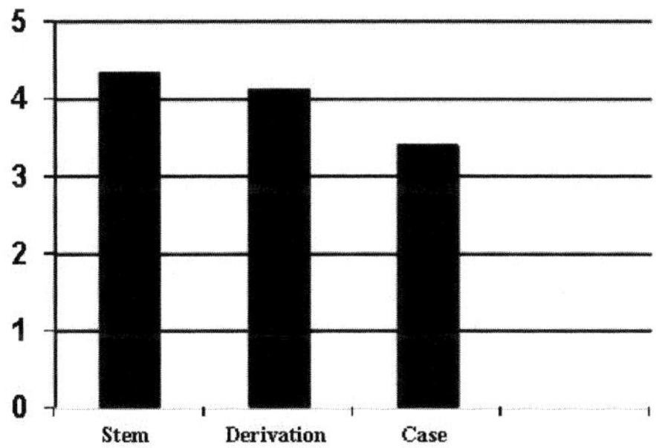

Fig. 2. Case marked nouns are more difficult to recall for Hungarian subjects (After Németh *et al.*, 2011).

They also found a cumulative memory constraint effect. "Suffixed words were more difficult to remember than stem words. ... not only was it easier for our participants to recall stem-words compared to one or two-suffix words, but the results followed a gradient. The more suffixes a word was composed of the more difficult it was to recall" (Németh *et al.*, 2011, p. 100).

Gergely and Pléh (1994) on the basis of similar data proposed a hypothesis regarding alternative processing strategies in two different language types. Regarding the relativity issue this implies, that speakers of grammatically very different languages do use identical general cognitive mechanisms or resources (such as working memory) but these identical mechanisms are differently tuned to the crucial issues of processing the given language type.

Table 4. Two language type dependent systems of sentence processing (Gergely and Pléh, 1995).

Characteristics	**Rich morphology**	**Poor morphology**
Overall	Analytic	Holistic
Grammatical decisions	Fast, local	Slow, global
Syntax	Non configurational	Configurational
Working memory stress	Within words	Phrase level

This approach claims a constrained relativity, unlike the approaches of the mid-20th Century. It merely suggests that the cross-linguistic differences lead to different strategies of interpretation. This sort of constrained relativity is a 'language-to-language use relativity'. It suggests that we rely on universal resources for sentence interpretation such as working memory, associative and rule based, automatic and effortful processes, the allocation of attention. These processes are flexibly used for different representational levels, and in a temporarily adaptive manner. As Hunt and Agnoli (1991) pointed out, similar differences also lead to differences in the use of different memory integrative mechanisms in sentence understanding. In configurational languages (É. Kiss, 1981, 1987) like English preservation of the actual sequential order is crucial on the level of words, while in non-configurational languages like Hungarian there is a need for strong sequence within words. Pléh and Sinkovits (2011) had shown in a sentence recognition study that the retention of order information is in fact rather flexible in Hungarian. Semantically irrelevant free word order variations are forgotten faster compared to English, while showing the adaptiveness if the system, order information that is relevant for contrastive focusing is preserved even after 40 seconds.

Unlike traditional relativity claims this constrained processing relativity does not imply that speakers of different languages would use their cognitive resources differently in non-linguistic tasks.

At the same time the locality and holism is not an absolute feature. While first fast decisions in Hungarian are based on local cues (case markers, and morphology in general), the results of these computations have to be fit into the wider full picture.

Brain Mechanisms and the Analytic/Holistic in Language

There are some interesting efforts to try to relate the language type issue to brain representation. Bever (1971) showed that the increase of effective left hemisphere dominance in language processes correlates with increasing use of the "first noun is the agent" strategy in sentence interpretation, showing a LH localization of an order based canonic form. One might have thought this to be a universal tendency. However, Bever already warned us that this means that the left hemisphere is related to the use of the most efficient parsing strategy in the given language. Starting from these ideas, in Hungarian, Pléh (1990) showed that children of the same age (4–6 years) displayed the opposite tendency; namely that with the increase of LH lateralization, a decrease was observed in the use of order-based strategies. It seems to be that the LH is tuned to the most valid cues of the given language. Therefore, the same brain areas recruited to support order-based strategies in English support morphology based strategies in Hungarian (Fedor *et al.*, 2009).

This is interestingly related to brain development. Between the age of 2 and 6, you see an increase in left hemisphere reliance on language processing, and an increase in left hemisphere dominance. This is measured by the dichotic listening task where from around 5 years a strong right ear/left brain advantage can be observed (Kimura, 2011). Moncrief (2015) showed this effect in normalized data for clinical purposes. This Left Hemisphere reliance in English is related to a more and more strict use of word order in interpreting sentences (Bever, 1971). Interestingly, in Hungarian it is the other way around. The more left brain localized a child is, the less the child is using word order and the more the child is only using case marking, as case marking is the most important grammatical feature in Hungarian. It seems to be that the LH is tuned to the most valid cues of the given language, or in the other terminology, to the canonic form. Therefore, the same brain areas recruited to support order-based strategies in English support morphology based strategies in Hungarian.

This is especially interesting, since recently several data indicate that there are differences in the ear advantages over 60 languages (Bless *et al.*, 2015), but this is rarely correlated with the actual language interpretation strategies. Some rather speculative claims made by Bichakjian (1999) suggest that this reliance on left hemisphere for language interpretation is the result of a move towards more analytic attitude towards language.

One crucial example is thematic role assignment, which seems to be done by the LH, but the cues used for this computation might differ greatly across languages. Investigating different cues across languages, Bornkessel and Schlesewsky (2006) argued that Broca's area supports thematic role assignment independent of the particular cue (word order, case marking, or animacy). They suggested that this region is responsible for mapping the linear sequence of cues regarding the position of a noun on a thematic hierarchy onto the thematic role assigned to each noun. In their view, "there are three stages in assigning structure to a sentence: (1) constituent structure building without relational interpretation, (2) argument role assignment via a restricted set of cross-linguistically motivated information types (e.g., case, animacy), and (3) completion of argument interpretation using information from further domains (e.g., discourse context, plausibility). This basic architecture is assumed to be universal" (ibid, p. 787). The cross-linguistic differences that are much emphasized by the processing type approaches show up in the second phase.

Clearly, there is a need to do systematic cross-linguistic comparisons using identical methods, both behaviorally and in regard to neuroscience data gathering, to reveal the exact nature of neural network activation in typologically different languages.

Friederici (2002) and Bornkessel-Schlesewsky *et al.* (2011) developed a line of research in using ERP patterns during sentence interpretation in a cross-linguistic frame as well. Mostly comparing Indo-European languages, as well as Turkish and Chinese, they proposed that the N400 is sometimes missing, namely when the functions are dependent on word order. Thus, the importance of word order is crucial in grammatical interpretation. Cross-linguistic differences, as indicated by much less analytical studies as well. In their interpretation, the rather than reflecting linguistic domains such as syntax and semantics, the ERP markers correspond to optimized interpretation strategies in the given languages.

Conclusions

There are two relevant proposals here. There are certainly processing differences in line with typological differences of languages. However, they are not of an all or none nature, and they are not related to East and West distinction. They are related to intricacies of the internal organization of the grammar of the given language which is a crucial demand on children to accommodate to. This processing type difference is only seemingly similar to the holistic and item based cognitive attitudes of processing proposed by Nisbett but it is not at all related to any East and West cultural differences, related to the internal issues of language.

- Languages differ in the language processing strategies they use, and this is related to the use of common resources according to language structure.
- Language shapes the selection between alternative representations, but is not the source of these representations. Some preferences are formed prelinguistically.
- We are not denying that language has an influence on cognitive functions but it has more modulating than determining influence. I personally do not believe that language sets up barriers for understanding speakers of other languages. It certainly makes certain things easier.

References

Bates, E. and MacWhinney, B. (1989) Functionalism & the Competition Model. In MacWhinney, B. and Bates, B. (Eds.), *The Crosslinguistic Study of Sentence Processing*. pp. 3-76, New York: Cambridge University Press.

Bever, T. G. (1971) The nature of the cerebral dominance in the speech behavior of the child and adult, in Huxley, T. and Ingram, E. (eds.): *Language Acquisition. Models and Methods,* London: Academic Press.

Bever, T. G. (2013) The biolinguistics of language universals: The next years. In: *Language Down the Garden Path: The Cognitive and Biological Basis for Linguistic Structures.* ed. by Sanz, M., Laka, I. and Tanenhaus, M. K. Oxford: Oxford University Press, pp. 374-402.

Bichakjian, B. H. (1999) Language evolution and the complexity criterion: Target article on language complexity, *Psycoloquy*, 10(033).

Bless, J. J., Westerhausen, R., Torkildsen, J. von K., Gudmundsen, M., Kompus, K. and Hugdahl, K. (2015) Laterality across languages: Results from a global dichotic listening study using a smartphone application. *Laterality, 20,* pp. 434-452.

Bornkessel, I. and Schlesewsky M. (2006) The extended argument dependency model: a neurocognitive approach to sentence comprehension across languages. *Psychol Rev. 113*(4):787-821.
Bornkessel-Schlesewsky, I., Kretzschmar, F., Tune, A., Wangb, L., Genc, S., Philipp, M., Roehm, D. and Schlesewsky, M. (2011) Think globally: Cross-linguistic variation in electrophysiological activity during sentence comprehension. *Brain & Language 117,* 133-152.
Boroditsky, L. (2001) Does Language Shape Thought?: Mandarin & English Speakers' Conception of Time. *Cognitive Psychology*, 43(1), 1-22.
Brown, R. W. and Lenneberg, E. H. (1954) A study in language and cognition, *J. Abnormal and Social Psychology 49,* 454-462.
Carroll, J. B. (ed.) (1956) Language, *Thought, & Reality: Selected Writings of Benjamin Lee Whorf.* MIT Press, Boston, Massachusetts.
Carroll, J. B. and Casagrande, J. B. (1958) The function of language classification in behavior, in Maccoby, E., Newcomb, F. and Hartley, E. (eds.): *Readings in Social Psychology,* pp. 18-31, New York: Holt.
Chan, H. M. and Yan, K. K. T. (2007) Is There a Geography of Thought for East-West Differences? Why or why not? *Educational Philosophy & Theory*, doi: 10.1111/j.1469-5812.2007.00346.
Chomsky, N. (1965) *Aspects of a Theory of Syntax,* Cambridge/Mass.: MIT Press.
Chomsky, N. (1966) *Cartesian Linguistics,* New York: Harcourt.
Chomsky, N. (1981) *Lectures on Government & Binding*, Mouton de Gruyter.
Chomsky, N. (1986) *Knowledge of Language*, New York: Praeger.
Chomsky, N. (1988) *Language & Problems of Knowledge*, Cambridge: MIT Press
Chua, H. F., Bol, J. E. and Nisbettt, R. E. (2005) Cultural variation in eye movements during scene perception, *Proceedings of the National Academy of Sciences, 102,* 12629-12633.
Cole, M. and Scribner, S. (1974) *Culture and Thought*, New York: Wiley.
Cooke, A., Zurif, E. B., DeVita, C., Alsop, D., Koenig, P., Detre, J., Gee, J., Pinango, M., Balogh, J. and Grossman, M. (2002) Neural basis for sentence comprehension: Grammatical and short-term memory components, *Human Brain Mapping, 15*, 80-94.
É. Kiss, K. (1981) Structural relations in Hungarian, a "free" word order language. *Linguistic Inquiry, 12*, 185-213.
É. Kiss, K. (1987) *Configurationality in Hungarian.* Budapest. Akadémiai Kiadó.
Fedor, A., Pléh, Cs. *et al.* (2009) What Are the Brain Mechanisms Underlying Syntactic Operations. In Bickerton, D. and Szathmáry, E. (eds.): *Biological Foundations & Origin of Syntax*. 299-321, Cambrige, MA: MIT Press.
Fodor, J. A. (1983) *The Modularity of Mind.* Cambridge, MA. MIT Press.
Fodor, J. A. (2008) *LOT 2: The Language of Thought Revisited.* Oxford University Press.
Friederici, A. D. T. (2002) Towards a neural basis of auditory sentence processing. *Trends Cogn Sci. 6,* 78-84.
Fuchs, C. and Robert, S. (eds., 1999) *Language Diversity and Cognitive Representations.* Amsterdam: Benjamins.
Gergely, G. (1991) *Free Word Order and Discourse Interpretation.* Budapest: Akadémiai Kiadó.
Gergely, Gy. and Pléh, Cs. (1994) Lexical Processing in an Agglutinative Language & the Organization of the Lexicon. *Folia Linguistica*, 28, 175-204.
Hirschfeld, L. A. (1994) Is the acquisition of social categories based on domain-specific competence or on knowledge transfer? In: Hirshfeld, L. A. and Gelman, S. A. (eds.): *Mapping the Mind. Domain Specificity in Cognition & Culture.* Cambridge, Mass.: pp. 201-233, Cambridge University Press.

Humboldt, W. von (1836/1999) *On Language. On the Diversity of Human Language Construction & its Influence on the Mental Development of the Human Species*. Ed. Michael Losonsky, Translated by Peter Heath. Cambridge: Cambridge University Press.

Hunt, E. and Agnoti, F. (1991) The Whorfian hypothesis: A cognitive psychology perspective, *Psychological Review,* 98, 377-389.

Ivády, R. E., Felhősi, G. and Pléh, Cs. (2008) A téri referenciakeretek változása az életkorral tipikusan fejlődő és Williams szindrómás gyerekeknél. 'Changes in spatial frames in typically developing an Williams syndrome children'. In Hungarian. *Magyar Pszichológiai Szemle, 63.* 213-250.

Kay, P. and Kempton, W. (1984) What is the Sapir-Whorf hypothesis?, *American Anthropologist 86*, 65-79.

Kimchi, R., Amishav, R. and Sulitzeanu-Kenan, A. (2009) Gender differences in global–local perception? Evidence from orientation and shape judgments. *Acta Psychologica 130,* 64-71.

Kimura D. (2011) From ear to brain. *Brain Cogn 76*(2):214-217.

Lantz, D. and Stefflre, V. (1964) Language and cognition revisited, *J. Abnormal and Social Psychology 69*, 472-481.

Lenneberg, E. H. (1953) Cognition in ethnolingustics. *Language, 29,* 463-471.

Levinson, S. C. (1996) Language and space. *Annual Review of Anthropology, 25,* 353-382.

Li, P. and Gleitman, S. (2002) Turning the tables: language and spatial reasoning. *Cognition, 83,* 265-294.

Li, P., Bates, E. and MacWhinney, B. (1993) Processing a language without inflections: A reaction time study of sentence interpretation in Chinese. *Journal of Memory & Language, 32,* 169-192.

Lucy, J. A. and Shweder, R. A. (1979) Whorf and his critics: Lingustic and nonlinguistic influences on color memory, *American Anthropologist 81*, 581-615.

MacWhinney, B. and Bates, E. (1989, eds.) *The crosslingulstic study of sentence processing.* Cambridge: Cambridge University Press.

MacWhinney, B., Pléh, Cs. and Bates, F. (1985) The devolopment of sentence interpretation in Hungarian, *Cognitive Psychology*, *17,* 178-209.

Menn, L. (2000) It's Time to Face a Simple Question: Why Is Canonical Form Simple? *Brain and Language, 71*,157 150.

Miller, G. A. and MacNeill, D. (1968) Psycholinguistics. In: Lindzey, G. and Aaronson, E. (eds.): *Handbook of social psychology. Vol. 3.* pp. 666-794, Reading, Mass.: Addison-Wesley.

Moncrief, D. (2015) Age- and Gender-Specific Normative Information from Children Assessed with a Dichotic Words Test. *J. Am. Acad. Audiol. 26*, 632-644.

Németh, D., Ivády, R. E., Guidac, A. Mihάltz, M., Peckhame, D., Krajcsi, A. and Pléh, Cs. (2011) The Effect of Morphological Complexity on Short-Term Memory Capacity. *Acta Linguistica Hungarica, 58,* 85-107.

Niemi, J., Laine, M. and Tuominen, J. (1994) Cognitive morphology in Finnish: Foundations of a new model. *Language and Cognitive Processes*, *9*, 423-446.

Nisbett, R. E. (2003) *The Geography of Thought: How Asians & Westerners Think Differently & Why*, New York: The Free Press.

Nisbett, R. E. and Masuda, T. (2003) Culture & point of view. *Proc. Natl. Acad. Sci. 100,* 11163-11175.

Nisbett, R. E. and Miyamoto, Y. (2005) The influence of culture: holistic versus analytic andperception. *Trends in Cognitive Sciences, 9,* 467-473.

Nisbett, R. E. *et al.* (2001) Culture and systems of thought: Holistic versus analytic cognition. *Psychol. Rev. 108,* 291–310.

Norenzayan, A. and Heine, S.J. (2005) Psychological universals: what are they & how can we know? *Psychol. Bull.* 131, 763-784.

Norenzayan, A. *et al.* (2002) Cultural preferences for formal versus intuitive reasoning. *Cogn. Sci. 26*, 653-684.

Pléh Cs. (1989) The development of sentence interpretation in Hungarian, in MacWhinney, B. and Bates, E. (eds.): *The Crosslinguistic Study of Sentence Processing,* Cambridge University Press 1989, 158-184.

Pléh Cs. (1990) Word order and morphophonological factors in the development of sentence understanding in Hungarian, *Linguistics 28,* 1449-1469.

Pléh, Cs. (2000) A relativizmus kérdései és a mai pszicholingvisztika. 'Issue of relativism in contemporary psycholinguistics'. Academy inaugural in Hungarian. In: Glatz Ferenc (szerk.): *Székfoglalók 1995-1998, Vol. III* Budapest: MTA, 2000.

Pléh, Cs. and Sinkovits, B. (2011) Word order and focusing effects in the memory representation of Hungarian sentences. *Acta Linguistica Hungarica, 58,* 120-133.

Rosch, E. (1975) Universals and cultural specifics in human categorization. In Brislin, R., Bochner, S. and Lonner W. (eds.): *Cross-cultural perspectives on learning.* pp. 177-206, New York: Saga.

Slobin, D. and Bever, Th. (1982) Children use canonical sentence schemes: A crosslinguistic study of word order & inflections, *Cognition 12*, 229-265.

Sperber, D. (1994) The modularity of thought & the epidemiology of representations. In: Hirshfeld, L. A. and Gelman, S. A. (eds.): *Mapping the Mind. Domain Specificity in Cognition & Culture.* Cambridge, pp. 39-67, Mass.: Cambridge University Press.

Sperber, D. (2000) Metarepresentations in an evolutionary perspective. In: Sperber, D. (ed.): *Metarepresentations.* New York: Oxford University Press.

Sperber, D. and Hirschfeld, L.A. (2004) The cognitive foundations of cultural stability & diversity. *Trends in Cognitive Sciences, 8,* 40-46.

Varnum, M. E. W., Grossmann, I. D. , Nisbett, R. E. and Kitayama, K. (2008) Holism in a European Cultural Context: Differences in Cognitive Style between Central & East Europeans & Westerners. *Journal of Cognition & Culture, 8*, 321-333.

Werner, H. and Wapner, S. (1949) Sensory-Tonic Field Theory of Perception, *Journal of Personality 18,* 88-107.

Whorf, B. (1939/1956) The relation of habitual thought & behavior to language. In J. B. Carroll (szerk.), *Language, thought, & reality: selected writings of Benjamin Lee Whorf*, pp. 134-159, Cambridge, MA: The MIT Press.

Whorf, B. (1941/1956) Language, mind, & reality. In J. B. Carroll (szerk.), *Language, thought, & reality: selected writings of Benjamin Lee Whorf*, pp. 134-159, Cambridge, MA: The MIT Press.

Witkin H. A., Lewis, H. B., Hertzman, M., Machover, K., Meissner, P. and Wapner, S. (1973) *Personality Through Perception: An experimental & clinical study*, Westport: Greenwood.

6 Searching for Unasked Questions: An Unfinished "East-West-exploration"

Ernst Pöppel[*,†,‡] and Yan Bao[†,*,§]

[*]Human Science Center and Institute of Medical Psychology, Ludwig-Maximilians-University, Munich, Germany
[†]School of Psychological and Cognitive Sciences, and Beijing Key Laboratory of Behavior and Mental Health, Peking University, Beijing, China
[‡]Ernst.Poeppel@med.uni-muenchen.de
[§]baoyan@pku.edu.cn

A Personal Remark about an Exploratory Frame

Coming from East and West, belonging to different age groups, representing different gender, having different mother tongues, in spite of this diversity, we, the two authors, experience enrichment in our work, although most of the time working together at a distance. We discover the unexpected, enjoy the challenges, have to deal also with frustrations. What happens in the exploratory frame when one works together "east of west, and west of east", geographically and metaphorically speaking? The way we think is different, the pace we work is different, the time perspectives are different; one is dedicated to the present, the other oriented to the future; and sometimes the time perspectives may turn around. The levels of discourse can be very different; he or she may focus on methodological aspects, she or he at the same time is seduced by speculations. One thinks that one question is most important, the other wants to follow another research trajectory. Most importantly, we discover perspectives of our own culture, which we never thought about before; we are confronted with our prejudices towards the other culture. Regular daily rituals for the one are disturbing for the other. Effortless actions become effortful in the new cultural environment. Given all these diversities and challenges, without trust, openness, respect and most importantly humor one cannot work together. In spite of all these problems, we share curiosity and enthusiasm to explore new research paths. There is a common desire to understand. In a broad frame of research interests there exists a common denominator searching for unasked questions and also hoping for unexpected answers; serendipity has to be harvested. Questions have to be discovered, and they sometimes jump into the mind when we just talk to each other, even at a distance with thousands of kilometers. The German poet Heinrich von Kleist (1777-1811) has characterized this phenomenon in an essay with a title that says it all, i.e., "Über die allmähliche Verfertigung der Gedanken beim Reden" (On the gradual development of thoughts while talking).

What are such questions? Beyond detailed questions in experimental design, methodological considerations, statistical procedures or technological challenges every researcher is confronted with, there are several general issues which provide the conceptual frame within which one acts. Here are some of our concerns: We use language in an unreflected way, as if a specific language is neutral with respect to what one wants to express; it is of course not. Or: Explanations of experimental results follow the principle of monocausality as if we are victims of Occam's razor to search for one and only one explanatory factor. Or: We think to have a brain is a necessary condition for solving problems, not appreciating that even unicellular organisms are quite smart. Or: We automatically assume that temporal processing of information is continuous neglecting the possibility of discrete time sampling, which in fact is the case. Or: In an unreflected way we assume to be embedded in a homogeneous perceptual space; we are not. Or, and this can even be considered as a scandal in our scientific endeavors: Why are we not bothered in cognitive neuroscience and psychology that we do not own a taxonomy or classification of function, not even asking that we do not have one? Only a taxonomy transforms entertaining research activities into real science.

The Double Language Trap

It would be a good idea, and it is a strong suggestion (which nobody will accept), that somebody working on "consciousness" (Pöppel, 1997), "attention" (Bao and Pöppel, 2007), "emotions" (Park *et al.*, 2015), "beauty" (Pöppel *et al.*, 2013; Zeki *et al.*, 2014), "reality" (Silveira *et al.*, 2012), "self" (Zaytseva *et al.*, 2014), or "belief" (Silveira *et al.*, 2015) should not be allowed to use these words for some time. This would of course require a lot of self-imposed mental discipline, but even if one cannot follow this suggestion one should try to express a thought in alternative ways. The use of these terms as *nouns* indicates the desire to "ontologize" neural or psychological processes, and nobody is free of this tendency. The philosopher and mathematician Bertrand Russell is said to have remarked once that we are justified to say that there is thinking, but we are not justified in saying that there is a *thing* which thinks, and that this thing is our mind. The human tendency to ontologize ("the" mind, "the" self, ...) has severe consequences for practical research. Activities in circumscribed areas of the brain as observed for instance with fMRI attract psychological attributions and interpretations that may reflect psychological confusion. An example: In well respected journals one can read (in different publications) that the insular cortex represents negative emotions, interoception, attentional shifts, pain, sex, craving, time perception, (and maybe others). This does not make sense. Presumably, a higher (or lower) neural activity in this area is necessary for these and maybe other cognitive functions, but the local neural activity is not a sufficient condition for the representation of complex psychological phenomena; these are represented in complex neural networks which have their own neural signatures for different functions, and local activities are just part of them. As an example: In comparing aesthetic and moral judgments (Avram *et al.*, 2003) it was shown that both types of judgments are characterized (as to be expected) by different neural networks, but that they share common components; in this particular case it was observed that the neural network for aesthetic judgments was embedded in the network of moral judgments; this observation implies that moral judgments contain an aesthetic component.

Besides the language (or better conceptual) trap of attributing complex psychological functions to local activities in the phrenological tradition going back for some 200 years, there is another trap which is usually overlooked in any scientific community or in society at large: Is it really true (as implicitly assumed) that it does not matter in which language ideas are expressed and experimental results in science are described? The practical experience of the two authors which probably mimics the experience of many others shows that this is not a trivial question: We cannot express ourselves the same way in English as we would do it in our mother tongues German or Chinese. Publishing scientific papers with colleagues whose first language is American English or English English (which are quite different), Chinese, Czech, German, Korean, Polish, Rumanian, and Russian as we have done over the years is always a unique linguistic challenge (Avram *et al.*, 2013,

2014; Han *et al.*, 2014; Mates *et al.*, 1994; Vedder *et al.*, 2015). We would write here a different manuscript if we would write in German or in Chinese. It is of course a great advantage that we can use a common language, but it would be a mistake to believe that the language is neutral with respect to the content to be communicated. The language does not only refer to the *way* content is communicated, but also to the *selection* of content itself. Thus, a language is not a neutral surface for the representation of thoughts. In addition, the connotation frame can also be very different: The English term "reality" refers both to an objective physically defined reality, but also to the subjective reality on an individual level; in German physical reality would refer to "Realität", and subjective reality to "Wirklichkeit". The lack of a verbal distinction could mask fundamental differences on the conceptual level.

Here is another example from our own research on temporal perception: The English "present" evokes other associations as the German "Gegenwart" or the Chinese "xian zai". The "present" refers to sensory re*present*ations, whereas "Gegenwart" has a more active flavor, as the component "warten" refers to "taking care of", or "waiting for something or somebody"; it is thus both past and future oriented. The Chinese "xianzai" is associated with something in its perceptual identity, and it implies a spatial reference indicating the "here" as the locus of experience, and it is also action oriented. Although the different semantic connections are usually not thought of explicitly, they still provide an implicit frame of reference (Pöppel and Bao, 2011; Zhou *et al.*, 2014), as research for instance on priming has shown (e.g., Lutz *et al.*, 2013; Silveira *et al.*, 2014). We cannot assume on the one hand that priming has on the implicit level an effect on cognitive processing, and believe on the other hand that it does not have an effect when using translated words in different languages.

"Monocausalities" as a Disease, and "Complementarity" as a Therapy

It does not happen too often that psychologists or cognitive neuroscientists discover a new disease, but we claim to have done so; the disease is "monocausalitis". Apparently, we are all victims of "Occam's razor" looking always for the simplest explanation, which however may be too simple; the simplest explanations are monocausal explanations. The fundamental philosophical sentence "nihil est sine ratione" (nothing is without reason) is easily interpreted as "nothing is without *one* reason"; it would be better to say "nihil est sine *rationibus*" (nothing is without *reasons*) to appreciate the complexity of what is observed.

To overcome this problem of misinterpreted simplicity one may adopt the thought pattern of complementarity from theoretical physics. To give just a few examples where this thought pattern applies: Perceptual processes as being reflected for instance in object recognition or face perception are necessarily both bottom-up *and* top-down (Zhou *et al.*, 2016); this does not mean that components of the process cannot be just this or that (transduction at the receptor level or neural mechanisms of attentional control), but they always have to come together to create content on the level of experience. Another example of complementarity as a thought pattern can be taken from the nature-nurture debate: There is of course evidence for genetic factors as for the experience of pain or pleasure, or of the phonetic repertoire in language; but there is also evidence for the importance of imprinting in early phases of life, i.e., the necessary selection or confirmation of partial sets of these genetically determined repertoires in different environments. Here epigenetics enters the field, and one is forced to conclude that it is both, the genetic endowment *and* the cultural frame that determine subjective realities (or the "Wirklichkeit"). It follows that complementarity would not only be a "thought pattern", but complementarity is a generative principle for cognitive processes; thus, monocausal explanations would be misleading.

This principle of complementarity applies also to research paradigms. There is a tendency in cognitive science to discard single case studies and to "allow" as a research paradigm only hypothesis testing using statistical procedures. But what is wrong with the paradigm to "harvest" single case studies in a complementary way? Most important discoveries have been made with single case studies and cognitive neuroscience and psychology would not exist without them. Single case studies have shaped psychology and brain science since its very beginning in the 19th century. Such studies provide the unique opportunity to answer previously unasked questions, and to discuss what is usually taken as self-evident in subjective experiences. Single case observations may lead to unexpected hypotheses which have remained silent before. Distinct lesions of the brain or observations with healthy subjects under unique circumstances can disentangle complex functions, for instance according to the principle of "double dissociation of function" (Milner and Teuber, 1968), and they open new windows to understand underlying mechanisms of cognitive processing (Martin and Hull, 2007). Cases like "tan-tan" (Broca, 1865), Henry M. (Scoville and Milner, 1957), or split-brain patients (Sperry, 1961) have opened new fields in the understanding of language, memory, or visual perception and their disturbances in different pathologies (Zaytseva *et al.*, 2015). Such exploratory studies may lead to new hypotheses for confirmatory studies using statistical methods. It is our impression that we have become blinded by statistics giving more credit to an analysis of variance or a principal component analysis than harvesting unique constellations of phenomena in a patient allowing unique insights into cognitive functions. Brain-injured patients are unfortunate experiments of nature; on the basis of their brain injuries a specific path of research can be opened that allows a better understanding of mental processes. Exploratory single case studies *and* confirmatory hypothesis-testing studies should be appreciated on equal level in a complementary way.

Unicellular Organisms as Models for Higher Cognition

Life started with unicellular organisms several billion years ago, and only several hundred million years ago multicellular organisms entered the world; this was the late start for the evolution of nervous systems. Multicellular organisms which move around in their physical environment require an information system between cells to process sensory input that concerns the entire organism, and to inform other cells about the internal state of the organism. Might it be conceivable that before multicellular organisms with such information systems or brains developed, unicellular organisms already had some functional competence similar to "high level" functioning as is usually attributed to organisms with brains? It has been suggested that for instance learning capacities are already implemented in such "low level" organisms (Lengeler *et al.*, 2000). It is inviting to take the famous statement of Dobzhansky (1973) that "nothing in biology makes sense, except in the light of evolution", and to look for potential similarities in functional competence in uni- and multicellular organisms "in the light of evolution". Our thoughts are of course speculative, but surprisingly on a conceptual level one can detect astonishing similarities in functional control between uni- and multicellular organisms. As a model organism we take the dinoflagellate *Gonyaulax polyedra* which has been extensively used in research on circadian rhythms (Roenneberg, 1996). This organism is responsible for the red tide as it emits light and moves vertically in the water at particular phases within 24 hours. It has been well established that circadian rhythms are a biological property on all levels of organismic complexity, i.e., from bacteria to primates including humans. The question is whether we can go beyond circadian rhythms to get insight into functional control and "cognitive competence". We do not claim that unicellular organisms are characterized by explicit knowledge as humans own it, but one has to keep in mind that many functions characterizing human behavior are controlled on an implicit level without explicit interference (Pöppel and Bao, 2011). Our body is smarter than what we know about our body.

A basic principle for regulation of life, maybe the most basic principle, is the maintenance of homeostasis or allostasis (to take into account the dynamic changes in environments to which organisms adapt). How can homeostasis be reached and maintained in unicellular organisms like *Gonyaulax polyedra*? To reach an optimal or better environment, goal-directed movements are necessary. These are not random movements; they have to be programmed in a certain direction in space. Prior to get the motor program going, several operations are necessary. The organism must have information where it is at present. This is made possible by molecular structures in the membrane that are sensitive to physical stimuli like in *Gonyaulax polyedra* to specific wavelengths of light. Thus, this organism can "see" although in a rather rudimentary sense. To measure light intensity at a specific wavelength at only one position in space is, however, not sufficient to inform the motor system of the organism in which direction it has to move. It is necessary to make a second measurement; only when at last two measurements are made, can they be compared to determine differences in light intensity and a potential gradient in flux which can serve as information for movement directions to be programmed. Thus, the mechanism of comparison is implemented already in these organisms; comparison as a "mental" operation is also characteristic for cognitive processes on a higher level. On an abstract level one has to conclude that the concept of relations between different organismic states is already established at the beginning if life.

When measuring light intensity at different spatial locations in order to compare them, the time difference between the two measurements has to be temporally limited; if the time difference would be too long the representation of the first measurement would have already faded away. Thus, one has to conclude that operative "time windows" already exist at this early stage of life. To allow a comparison between successive states it is necessary that the first measurement is still available which implies a specific memory function. If the two measurements give similar values, the movement system does not get reliable information and moves randomly like in typical search behaviors of organisms with brains. Thus, comparisons resulting in equal or different light intensities determine goal-directed or random movements. It follows that the concept of a threshold is already critical on this organismic level. In the next step, if the two "percepts" based on the measurements of light intensity are different, the organism can make a choice and a decision in which direction to move.

As indicated movements are necessary to search for environmental conditions where homeostatis can be reached. This implies that on the way to a new location the homeostatic state is not yet reached; this furthermore implies the existence of an evaluation system in the organism like for instance still being "hungry". Goal-directed movements to obtain better conditions for homeostasis lead to the conclusion that a better organismic state is anticipated. Thus, the organism must own already an implicit concept of time as otherwise such anticipation would not be possible. Finally, when the optimal location is reached another mechanism has come into play which can be related to the reafference principle (von Holst and Mittelstaedt, 1950). When programming a movement towards a better environment, a copy is made of this program, the "efference copy"; when a new location is reached, the efference copy is compared with the reafference (the sensory information collected from the external world). When the two match, the organism "knows" that the goal is reached. This operation of comparing efference copy and reafference provides also a monitoring system of being either still underway or having reached the goal.

Looking at all these different necessary operations to establish and maintain a homeostatic state, i.e., perception, comparison, evaluation, choice and decision, movement control, anticipation, time windows, memory, there is not much to add if one describes cognitive functions in high level organisms with brains. What seems to be missing in unicellular organisms is "theory of mind", i.e., to have an explicit representation of knowledge, (and even that cannot be claimed with certainty). This conceptual comparison of functional competence between unicellular and multi-cellular organisms and its suspected similarity leads to a further conclusion: If during the evolutionary process equivalent functional competences have developed in organisms with and without brains, it is suggested that physical characteristics of the world provide the option space for developments or even dictate specific evolutionary trajectories not only for bodily features but also for behavioral strategies to obtain and maintain optimal internal states.

Is Visual Space Homogeneous or Segmented?

It is usually taken for granted that our "visual world" (Gibson, 1950) is characterized by homogeneity matching physical principles. We hypothesize, however, that homogeneity of visual space has to be created. How do we come to such a hypothesis? In detailed measurements of increment threshold throughout the visual field to determine a two-dimensional sensitivity map (Pöppel and Harvey, 1973), one subject (E.P.) observed that the apparent brightness of threshold stimuli varied systematically throughout the visual field. Threshold targets at different eccentricities did not have (as to be expected in the tradition of classical psychophysics) the same apparent brightness, but they appeared brighter in the periphery of the visual field compared to the foveal and perifoveal regions. This observation was rather counter-intuitive (and still is), as one would expect that at threshold for any location in the visual field the apparent brightness should be the same. Based on this initial observation, apparent brightness for supra-threshold targets was studied systematically both under photopic and scotopic adaptation conditions (Zihl *et al.*, 1980). The results indicated that the apparent brightness of supra-threshold stimuli corresponded to their physical intensity, (however, for photopic adaptation conditions, only). This observation implies that the "operating range" between threshold brightness and supra-threshold brightness is getting continuously smaller for more peripheral visual targets.

This phenomenon of brightness constancy throughout the visual field can be considered as the functional basis for its homogeneity on the phenomenal level. Where in the afferent stream of visual information processing might be brightness constancy and as a consequence homogeneity of the visual field be created? For ecological reasons one can assume that this process should be localized as early as possible, i.e., already in the retina. If targets with equal physical brightness would appear darker in the periphery of the visual field as one would predict if apparent brightness is determined by multiples of threshold values (using traditional psychophysical reasoning), their chance to be detected would be worse compared to targets closer to the visual axis. Using a teleonomic argument it is in the interest for optimal attentional control that independent of where something will appear in the visual field, it should have equal probability to be detected. Only then spatial attention can be drawn without bias to any position in the visual field, and information appearing in the periphery of the visual field would not be neglected; only then can saccadic eye movements be programmed appropriately. As saccadic eye movements are elicited by stimuli which are projected to the superior colliculus in the midbrain, the compensatory mechanism to allow equal probability should be prior to the collicular processing stage. Thus, the creation of constancy of brightness should be implemented already in the retina. In this case equal probability of responses towards unexpected visual stimuli anywhere in the visual field would be guaranteed.

How could this paradoxical situation be overcomed already at the retina, i.e., compensating for the decrease of sensitivity towards the periphery by creating contours of equal brightness throughout the visual field? The hypothesis is forwarded that more peripheral ganglion cells in the retina and their surrounding network are characterized by different summation properties compared to near-fovea ganglion cells; instead of a (more) sigmoid gain function in perifoveal regions, ganglion cells in the periphery should show a non-linearity of summation at threshold; the firing rate of retinal ganglion cells "jumps" from the level of the spontaneous firing frequency "instantaneously", i.e., with very short latency, to a higher level of firing frequency. This compensatory mechanism with different summation properties would explain why the apparent brightness is higher for peripheral targets. To the best of our knowledge summation properties of ganglion cells in the primate retina including the far periphery of the visual field have not been investigated in detail, although promising results have been obtained from the cat retina (Roenneberg and Pöppel, 1985). It should be noted that for the plateau region extending approximately between 10 to 35 degrees eccentricity along the horizontal meridian, and from 10 to 20 degrees eccentricity along the vertical meridian (Pöppel and Harvey, 1973), the same gain functions would be expected.

If the phenomenon of constancy of brightness is already implemented at the retinal level, another problem would also be solved at a very early processing stage, i.e., that the apparent brightness is the same for the two halves of the visual field, although they are represented in different hemispheres of the brain. In that case no intercallosal interactions between the different hemispheric representations would be necessary with respect to equalizing brightness as they are getting the same information anyway. Furthermore, a top-down mechanism could be spared, i.e., that the apparent homogeneity of the visual field is thought to match directly the physical parameters of optical stimuli because common sense indicates that the "visual world" (Gibson, 1950) does not show any inhomogeneity with respect to lightness under photopic conditions.

Constancy of brightness throughout the visual field is also crucial for the control of visual attention. It has been shown with the experimental paradigm of "inhibition of return" (IOR) that spatial attention to perifoveal and peripheral visual targets is controlled by different mechanisms (Bao and Pöppel, 2007). This eccentricity effect is resistant to practice (Bao *et al.*, 2011), and it cannot be explained by the magnification factor (Bao *et al.*, 2013a). It has been proven to be a genuine phenomenon which is substantiated also by observations using imaging technologies, i.e., fMRI (Lei *et al.*, 2012), and MEG (Zhou *et al.*, 2010). Although being controlled by different neural mechanisms, they share the same time window (Bao *et al.*, 2013c; Bao *et al.*, 2015) which guarantees together with constancy of brightness throughout the visual field a unified spatio-temporal platform for visual processing. We conclude that the homogeneity of visual space has to be constructed for the purpose of equal probability to detect visual targets and to draw visual attention to them in an unbiased way.

Is Time Discrete, or is Time Continuous?

In 1868 the Dutch physiologist Karl Donders developed the concept that differences in reaction times for defined experimental protocols can be used to analyze cognitive processes. This method of chronometric analyses is applied probably in every psychological laboratory in the world, but it suffers from the unquestioned assumption, that "time" (temporal processing) is a continuous variable. But this is the question: Is "time" in the brain represented as a continuous function, (if it is a function at all)? If one analyzes temporal perception it is important to acknowledge that we cannot perceive "time" itself, but that we refer on the perceptual level to events. Looking at the neural representation of events in its complexity, the construction and maintenance of conscious phenomena is rather enigmatic. How can we get closer to deal with the challenges of event creation and the establishment of conscious content? We believe to look in some detail into temporal processing and what we refer to as "temporal windows" (Bao *et al.*, 2015), and to discuss the question whether "time" actually is processed continuously, or whether it is not necessary to assume a discrete strategy which indeed appears to be the case for a low level of information processing. Apparently the nervous system has developed strategies in evolution to overcome inherent problems for instance due to the complexity of the physical world. Where do these problems come from? There are several sources giving rise to complexity, uncertainty or even disarray of neuronal information, i.e., the physics of stimuli, biophysical constraints in the transduction of stimuli, and their central anatomical representation.

One source of uncertainty comes from stimulus transduction which is principally different in the sense modalities like audition or vision, taking less than one millisecond in the auditory system and more than twenty milliseconds in the visual system. Thus, auditory and visual information arrive at different times in central processing areas of the brain. To overcome uncertainty becomes more complicated by the fact that the transduction time in the visual modality is also flux-dependent, i.e., that objects in visual space with less flux require more transduction time at the receptor surface in the retina. Thus, to see an object with areas of different brightness or to see somebody talking, different temporal availabilities of local activities within the visual modality, and similarly different local activities across the two involved modalities have to be overcome. If in addition somatosensory information has to be integrated also to identify an object and to maintain its perceptual identity, the integrating systems in the brain are confronted with even more temporal challenges as the transduction time in the somatosensory system again is different. Obviously, challenges of integration for different sensory channels become even bigger on higher levels of processing.

For inter-sensory integration, besides biophysical problems as given by the transduction times, also physical problems have to be considered. The distance of objects which are caught by attention is obviously never predetermined; anything can appear unexpectedly at any position in space with varying distances. Thus, the speed of sound (not of light) becomes a critical factor for the central availability of information. Approximately at a distance of ten meter transduction time in the retina (under optimal conditions of brightness) corresponds to the time the sounds requires to travel to the recipient. Up to this "horizon of simultaneity" auditory information arrives earlier in the brain; beyond this horizon, visual information is earlier. Again, there must be some kind of mechanism in the neuro-cognitive machinery which solves this problem of temporal uncertainty and unpredictability.

Besides biophysical and physical aspects there is a further problem of complexity which is introduced by the specific architecture of our brain (Nauta and Feirtag, 1986). As is suggested by neuro-anatomical studies there must be a considerable degree of divergence in the thalamo-cortical projections, i.e., each neuron innervating many cortical neurons (e.g., Gilbert and Wiesel, 1985). This means that local information is spread out over a wide array of receptive neurons, and because of the different transmission times along the axons of these neurons, local information characterizing an object is not only distributed spatially in a network of neurons but it is also diluted over time. The central neuronal representation is nothing like a passive mirror which veridically reflects what is going on in the world. Within the neuronal machinery events or objects are ill-defined and show a high degree of uncertainty both spatially and temporally.

How can this complex situation be overcome, how can the uncertainty be minimized? There is quite a lot of evidence with qualitatively different experimental paradigms that such a mechanism of complexity reduction may be at work. It is suggested that the problems mentioned above can be overcome if the nervous system uses stimulus triggered neuronal oscillations as derived for instance from experiments on choice reaction time (Pöppel, 2009). One period of such an oscillation is hypothesized to represent the functional basis of an elementary integration unit within which temporally and spatially distributed information is automatically related to each other and integrated into a unit. Such units or system states are insensitive to the exact temporal occurrence of input data. Thus, they are a-temporal and provide integration intervals within which information is treated as co-temporal. As a consequence "time" as conceived of in classical physics as a continuous variable does not exist. For complexity reduction the brain leaves Newtonian physics behind and uses "time windows" within which continuity of time is discarded as all information is treated as being simultaneous.

This adds up to the conclusion that temporal processing on this level must be of discrete nature (Bao *et al.*, 2013b). Successive "time windows" (Bao *et al.*, 2015) are necessary to create an operative basis for cognitive processing. This concept of discrete temporal processing continues to work in other temporal domains as well. On a next level of complexity reduction the primordial events represented in discrete system states are linked together, and another time window is created on a higher level of processing. What is the experimental evidence? If subjects have to reproduce the duration of either an auditory or a visual stimulus, one observes close to veridical reproductions with small temporal variance up to two to three seconds, and large errors of reproduction with a tendency for a shorter reproduction for longer intervals. It appears as if short intervals can be kept as a unit in working memory, while longer intervals temporally disintegrate. Temporal integration can also be studied by subjective accentuation of metronome beats. One of the founding fathers of experimental psychology, Wundt (1911), pointed out that temporal grouping of successive stimuli has a temporal limit of approximately two and a half seconds. In such a metronome task the subject imposes a subjective structure onto identical physical events. If auditory stimuli-like click sounds follow each other with an inter-stimulus interval of for instance one second, it is easy to impose a subjective structure by giving a subjective accent to every second of the stimuli. If, however, the temporal interval between the stimuli becomes too long (for instance 5 seconds), one is no longer capable to impose such a subjective temporal structure. The two sequential stimuli no longer can be united into one percept, i.e., temporal binding for temporally adjacent stimuli is no longer possible because they are represented within successive time windows.

Furthermore, the spontaneous alteration rate in the two sensory modalities, i.e., vision and audition, suggest that after an exhaust period of two to three seconds attentional mechanisms are elicited that open the sensory channels for new information; if the sensory stimulus remains the same, the alternative interpretation will gain control being consciously represented. Metaphorically speaking, every two to three seconds, the endogenously generated question arises “what is new”, and with unusual stimuli such as ambiguous material the temporal eigen-operations of the brain are unmasked.

Recent research on “inhibition of return” (IOR) gives also important access to temporal control of attention (Bao and Pöppel, 2007). If one attends to a specific position in the visual field, and attention has to be redrawn to this position after a short interruption, reaction time is prolonged as if a return is “inhibited”. The time window of such an inhibited return is, however, limited to approximately three seconds (Bao *et al.*, 2013c). Further support for a time window of two to three seconds comes from new experiments using the mismatch negativity (MMN) as an indicator (Wang *et al.*, 2015); in an oddball paradigm MMN is the neural response to rare stimuli in a regular temporal sequence of stimuli. If different interstimulus intervals (ISI) are employed covering a range from 1.5 to 6.0 seconds, the MMN has the highest amplitude for midline structures of the brain at about three seconds; this phenomenon reflects an endogenous temporal modulation of temporal sensitivity at the cortical mantle.

As the different experiments and observations employ qualitatively different paradigms covering perceptual processes in audition and vision, cognitive evaluations, movement control, speech, cultural artifacts, mnemonic representation, perceptual accentuation or temporal integration, it can be concluded that temporal integration in the range of two to three seconds represents a general principle of the neuro-cognitive machinery. This universal integration process is automatic and pre-semantic, i.e., it is not determined by what is processed, but it creates a time window within which conscious activities can be implemented. The time window is not created by sensory input, but it is used for sensory input (Pöppel and Bao, 2014). It has to be stressed that this time window should not be understood as a physical constant but as a temporal operating range endogenously generated. This time window on a higher processing level adds up to the conclusion that temporal processing is discrete. From a theoretical point of view this has even to be expected as the identity of percepts or thoughts has to be kept over some time, but not forever, i.e., the identity has to be limited to a temporal interval (Pöppel, 2010).

Although for the sake of complexity reduction temporal processing must be discrete, "time" can also be considered as being continuous (as it is usually implicitly assumed). However, subjective continuity of time is implemented on another conceptual level. It can be argued that the semantic connection between the content of what is represented in successive time windows results in the "illusion" of continuous time. This is, however, a necessary illusion in which subjective time is mapped onto time as defined in classical physics. Thus, we suggest the concept of complementarity as a generative principle in cognitive science: On a "lower" or operational level, time has to be discrete for reasons of complexity reduction of information and maintenance of identity of percepts and thoughts, but on a "higher" level of reasoning time is conceived of being continuous.

Searching for a Taxonomy of Functions

It may come as a surprise, if neuroscientists and psychologists say about their own scientific field that it misses the most important characteristics of a science, but this unfortunately is the case: We actually do not have a taxonomy or classification of those functions which we study. Biology or chemistry became accepted sciences after such taxonomies had been developed, but our science does not have a generally accepted classificatory system. Even worse: We do not even know that we do not have it. Instead of a taxonomy which might be accepted by the majority of the researchers and, thus, would be the basis of a joint endeavour, there are a number of conceptual models that determine the way research can be done (Pöppel and Ruhnau, 2011). It should be stressed, however, that within their frames of reference, these models certainly have been quite useful and successful, but what has to be stressed also is the fact that this success is limited to answers of questions which are necessarily defined by the constraints of the models and, thus, lack generality with respect to a general understanding of cognitive processes.

One such conceptual model is oriented towards physics, and "psychophysics" as it was developed some 150 years ago is still present and actually quite dominant in the rational conjectures about an understanding of cognitive mechanisms (Stevens, 1975). One of the rare mathematical descriptions of psychological phenomena has been formulated within this framework, i.e., the power law: The logarithm of the subjective intensity is proportional to the logarithm of the physical intensity multiplied by a factor which specifies the perceptual modality; the factors happen to vary approximately between 0.3 (as for brightness) and 3.0 (as for pain). From a psychological point of view this conceptual model of functions is based on a physical description of the world, and the task of the researcher is to map the physical world onto the world of subjective representations by defining objective expressions of such relationships. Without question, this approach has been successful as for instance in the adaption-level theory by Helson (1964) which provides a formal account on internal reference systems: Whenever stimuli are characterized by different intensities we are building up a cognitive matrix with a central reference point which corresponds to the geometric mean of the stimuli processed. But something is missing with respect to subjective reality (in German "Wirklichkeit") as not everything in human experience can be included into this conceptual frame; it is too limited a category system excluding subjective phenomena like emotions which are rather unlikely to be mapped onto the physical world.

Another conceptual model is based on the belief that cognitive phenomena are directly represented in human language. This linguistic model is deeply rooted in Western culture, like in the thinking of René Descartes (1637). Within this concept it is believed that humans can master the world and navigate through life only with explicit knowledge and this knowledge is veridically represented in language. The underlying hypothesis about human nature has had an important influence in modern times on the development of artificial intelligence with its concept of "physical symbol systems", but as Dreyfus (1979) has pointed out, it had to fail, in particular as the bodily aspect of human nature had been neglected.

That the linguistic model cannot include the entirety of what makes humans human, can also be derived from an analysis of the different knowledge systems (Pöppel and Bao, 2011). We have to distinguish at least three knowledge systems. In addition to explicit knowledge whose importance of course cannot be denied, our mental apparatus is characterized by implicit or tacit knowledge, and also by pictorial knowledge. How can the three modes of knowledge be characterized? Explicit knowledge is information with meaning which usually can be expressed verbally. Explicit knowledge is consciously available and it can be communicated using symbol systems like language. When something is forgotten, it can be recovered from documents, i.e., explicit knowledge is represented in encyclopedia, textbooks or nowadays in the internet. Explicit knowledge is accumulated by learning and this learning results in a corpus of semantic knowledge. The second mode of knowledge refers to implicit knowledge, i.e., to what we can do without being able to explicitly indicate how or why we are doing it. The difference between explicit and implicit knowledge might be characterized by two statements, one going back to Socrates who said: "I know that I do not know". Restating this sentence to characterize implicit knowledge, one could say: "I do not know that I know". An expression of implicit knowledge is also ritualized knowledge that characterizes daily activities. What one refers to as intuition is also an expression of implicit knowledge. The third mode of knowledge is visual knowledge, and it can be subdivided into different domains as being represented for instance in episodic memory (mnemonic visual knowledge), or topological visual knowledge, as it is seen in geometric figures, visual models, diagrams or histograms, and that allows the construction of maps; and visual knowledge is represented most powerfully also in art (e.g., Pöppel *et al.*, 2013; Silveira *et al.*, 2012, 2014). Mnemonic visual knowledge is anchored in the past and episodes that have some personal relevance are stored in memory for a lifetime.

Thus, topological visual knowledge is qualitatively different from mnemonic visual knowledge; whereas the latter refers to natural images, topological visual knowledge is based on visual abstractions.

Taken together it becomes obvious that the linguistic model represents only a partial set of what goes on in the human mind and can, thus, not be taken as a taxonomy of functions. A derivative of the linguistic model is a common sense model based on the unreflected use of language, and one could also refer in this case to a "textbook model". Humans have a natural tendency to ontologize their mental environment by the invention and uncritical use of words (see above). Looking at textbooks the titles of the chapters imply a classification of functions. One implication of these different entries is that they represent independent mental phenomena like perception, memory, emotion, attention, motivation, action, intelligence, consciousness, etc. Fact is that this textbook model actually dominates the scientific activities in this field. One rather unfortunate consequence of this model is that some researchers actually try to find the site of consciousness in the brain not realizing that such terms are rather new cultural inventions, and that they also have sometimes not the same meaning in different languages. We would like to indicate one other problem of this unreflected model, i.e., the conceptual mistake if one treats perception and attention on the same categorical level. Perception refers to content, attention refers to the way how content is created; it is necessary to logically distinguish between content and logistical functions of the neural systems (Pöppel, 1989; Bao and Pöppel, 2012). And there other models which have their value within their own frame of reference, and they have been certainly quite useful to gain more insight into human nature, like the psychoanalytical model (Freud, 1932) or the ethological model (Lorenz, 1943), but again only a partial set of the mental machinery of humans is taken into account.

There may, however, be a way out of the problem not having a taxonomy, i.e., if one adopts a hybrid approach and includes knowledge from neuropsychology. A "hybrid model" refers to the idea that the accumulated knowledge from the different models should be integrated. The neuropsychological model refers to the unique opportunity provided by observations with neurological or psychiatric patients (e.g., Luria, 1968, 1973; Milner and Teuber, 1968). The loss of functions in defined patient groups allows a classification of functions, as the loss of a function proves its existence; only what exists can be lost.

In an attempt to develop a taxonomy or more reliable classification of functions on the basis of neuropsychological observations (Pöppel,

1989), a distinction has been made between two functional domains which refer to the content of our experiences ("What"-functions) and to logistical functions ("How"-functions). These domains are differentially open to imprinting or epigenetic selections during ontogenetic processes. Anthropological universals as reflected in attentional modulation, activation or temporal organization of mental processes are rather robust against environmental factors, whereas "what"-functions like perceptions, memories, emotional evaluations, volitions or value systems are open to cultural imprinting (Bao and Pöppel, 2012). Content functions appear to be associated with the integrity of spatial modules within networks of the brain, whereas logistical functions are of a more distributed nature throughout neuronal networks. But it has to be stressed that the functional integrity of separate modules is just a necessary but not sufficient condition for cognitive processes. As indicated above a real danger in neuroscience and psychology is to fall into the trap of phrenology by associating uncritically the neuronal activity in a circumscribed area of the brain with high level cognitive processes. The interconnectivity of neuronal systems has always to be appreciated which as a consequence leads to the conclusion that there is never any independence of processing between different modules. The real challenge in our research is to formulate in mathematical language the specific networks of defined subjective states; the methodological possibilities with imaging technology like fMRI (Logothetis, 2008) are now available to reach this goal. Using a hybrid approach with vertical interdisciplinarity, i.e., from the cellular to the organismic and even social level, finally a reliable and generally accepted taxonomy of functions might be in sight.

Acknowledgments

Research referred to in this chapter was supported by German Research Foundation (DFG), German Federal Ministry of Education and Research (BMBF), Bavarian Research Foundation (BFS), Hanns-Seidel-Foundation (HSS), German Academic Exchange Service (DAAD), and National Natural Science Foundation of China (No. 31371018 and 91120004).

References

Avram, M., Gutyrchik, E., Bao, Y., Pöppel, E., Reiser, M. and Blautzik, J. (2013) Neurofunctional correlates of aesthetic and moral judgments: Equal but not the same. *Neuroscience Letters* 534, 128-132.

Avram, M., Hennig-Fast, K., Bao, Y., Pöppel, E., Reiser, M., Blautzik, J., Giordano, J. and Gutyrchik, E. (2014) Neural correlates of moral judgments in first- and third-person perspectives: implications for neuroethics and beyond. *BMC Neuroscience*, 15:39.

Bao, Y., Sander, T., Trahms, L., Pöppel, E., Lei, Q. and Zhou, B. (2011) The eccentricity effect of inhibition of return is resistant to practice. *Neuroscience Letters, 500*, 47-51.

Bao, Y., Lei, Q., Fang, Y., Tong, Y., Schill, K., Pöppel, E. and Strasburger, H. (2013a) Inhibition of Return in the Visual Field: The Eccentricity Effect is Independent of Cortical Magnification. *Experimental Psychology* 60, 425-431.

Bao, Y. and Pöppel, E. (2007) Two spatially separated attention systems in the visual field: evidence from inhibition of return. *Cognitive Processing* 8, 37-44.

Bao, Y. and Pöppel, E. (2012) Anthropological universals and cultural specifics: Conceptual and methodological challenges in cultural neuroscience. *Neuroscience and Biobehavioral Reviews* 36, 2143-2146.

Bao, Y., Pöppel, E., Wang, L., Lin, X., Yang, T., Avram, M., Blautzik, J., Paolini, M., Silveira, S., Vedder, A., Zaytseva, Y. and Zhou, B. (2015) Synchronization as a biological, psychological and social mechanism to create common time: A theoretical frame and a single case study. *PsyCh Journal* 4, 243–254 DOI: 10.1002/pchj.119.

Bao, Y., Szymaszek, A., Wang, X., Oron, A., Pöppel, E. and Elzbieta Szelag (2013b) Temporal order perception of auditory stimuli is selectively modified by tonal and non-tonal language environments. *Cognition* 129, 579-585.

Bao, Y., Wang, Z., Liang, W., Wang, Y., Pöppel, E. and Li, H. (2013c) Inhibition of return at different eccentricities in the visual field share the same temporal window. *Neuroscience Letters* 534, 7-11.

Broca, P. (1865) Sur le siège de la faculté du langage articulé. *Bull. Soc. Anthropol. 6*, 337-393.

Descartes, R. (1637, 1990) *Discours de la Méthode (Discourse on method).* Hamburg, Felix Meiner.

Dobzhansky, T. (1973) Nothing in biology makes sense, except in the light of evolution. *The American Biology Teacher, 35*, 125-129.

Donders, F. C. (1868 / 1969) On the speed of mental processes. *Acta Psychologica*, 30, 412-431.

Dreyfus, H. L. (1979) *What Computers can't Do. The Limits of Artificial Intelligence.* New York, Harper and Row.

Freud, S. *Neue Folge der Vorlesungen zur Einführung in die Psychoanalyse. (New series of lectures as introduction into psychoanalysis)*, Gesammelte Werke, Band 15, S. Fischer Verlag, Frankfurt, 3. Aufl. 1961 (orig. 1932).

Gibson, J. J. (1950) *The perception of the visual world.* The Riverside Press, Cambridge, Massachusetts, USA.

Gilbert, C. D. and Wiesel, T. N. (1985) Intrinsic connectivity and receptive field properties in visual cortex. *Vision Research, 25*, 365-374. doi:10.1016/0042-6989(85)90061-6.

Han, K. H., Zaytseva, Y., Bao, Y., Kim, H. T., Chung, S. Y., Kim, J. W. and Pöppel, E. (2014) Impairment of the vocal expression of emotions in patients with Alzheimer's Disease. *Frontiers in Aging Neuroscience*, doi:10.3389/fnagi.2014.00101.

Helson, H. (1964) *Adaptation-Level Theory. An Experimental and Systematic Approach to Behavior.* New York, Harper and Row.

Holst, E. v. and Mittelstaedt, H. (1950) Das Reafferenzprinzip (The reafference principle). *Naturwissenschaften* 37, 464-476.

Lei, Q., Bao, Y., Wang, B. and Gutyrchik, E. (2012) fMRI correlates of inhibition of return in perifoveal and peripheral visual field. *Cognitive Processing, 13 (Suppl.)*, S223-S227. doi:10.1007/s10339-012-0487-3.

Lengeler, J. W., Müller, B. S. and di Primo, F. (2000) Neubewertung kognitiver Leistungen im Lichte der Fähigkeiten einzelliger Lebewesen. (New evaluation of cognitive functions

in the light of competences of unicelluar organisms). *Kognitionswissenschaft* 8, 160-178.
Logothetis, N. (2008) What we can and what we cannot do with fMRI. *Nature* 453, 869-878.
Lorenz, K. (1943) Die angeborenen Formen möglicher Erfahrung (Innate forms of possible experience). *Zeitschrift für Tierpsychologie* 5, 235-409.
Luria, A. R. (1968) *The Mind of a Mnemonist. A Little Book about a Vast Memory*. New York, Basic Books.
Luria, A. R. (1973) *The Working Brain. An Introduction to Neuropsychology*. Basic Books, New York.
Lutz, A., Nassehi, A., Bao, Y., Pöppel, E., Sztrókay, A., Reiser, M., Fehse, K. and Gutyrchik, E. (2013) Neurocognitive processing of body representations in artistic and photographic images. *NeuroImage* 66, 288-292.
Martin, R. and Hull, R. (2007). The case study perspective on psychological research. In R. J. Sternberg, H. L. Roediger III and D. F. Halpern (Eds.): Critical Thinking in Psychology, pp. 90-109, Cambridge. Cambridge University Press.
Mates, J., Müller, U., Radil, T. and Pöppel, E. (1994) Temporal integration in sensorimotor synchronization. *Journal of Cognitive Neuroscience* 6, 332-340.
Milner, B. and Teuber, H.-L. (1968) Alteration of perception and memory in man: Reflections on methods. In: L. Weiskrantz (Ed.) *Analysis of Behavioral Change*, pp. 268-375, Harper and Row, New York.
Nauta, W. J. H. and Feirtag, M. (1986) *Fundamental Neuroanatomy*. Freeman & Co., New York.
Park, M., Gutyrchik, E., Welker, L., Carl, P., Pöppel, E., Zaytseva, Y., Meindl, T., Blautzik, J., Reiser, M. and Bao, Y. (2015) Sadness is unique: Neural Processing of Emotions in Speech Prosody in Musicians and Non-musicians. *Frontiers in Human Neuroscience* 2015, doi: 10.3389/fnhum.2014.01049.
Pöppel, E. (1989) Taxonomy of the Subjective: An Evolutionary Perspective. In: J. W. Brown (Ed.): *Neuropsychology of Visual Perception*. Lawrence Erlbaum Associates, Hillsdale, N.J., USA, 219-232.
Pöppel, E. (1997) Consciousness versus states of being conscious. *Behavioral and Brain Sciences* 20, 155-156.
Pöppel, E. (2009) Pre-semantically defined temporal windows for cognitive processing. *Philosophical Transactions of the Royal Society B* 363, 1887-1896.
Pöppel, E. (2010) Perceptual identity and personal self: Neurobiological reflections: In: Tomasz Maruszewski, Malgorzata Fajkowska and Michael M. Eysenck (Eds.) *Personality from biological, cognitive, and social perspectives*. Eliot Werner Publications, Clinton Corners, New York, 75-82.
Pöppel, E., Avram, M., Bao, Y., Graupmann, V., Gutyrchik, E., Lutz, A., Park, M., Reiser, M., Russell, E., Silveira, S., Smigielski, L., Szymanski, Y. and Zaytseva, Y. (2013) Sensory processing of art as a unique window into cognitive mechanisms: Evidence from behavioral experiments and fMRI studies. *Procedia – Social and Behavioral Sciences* 86, 10-17.
Pöppel, E. and Bao, Y. (2011) Three modes of knowledge as basis for intercultural cognition and communication: A theoretical perspective In: Shihui Han and Ernst Pöppel (eds.): *Culture and Neural Frames of Cognition and Communication*, Springer-Verlag, Heidelberg, 215-231.
Pöppel, E. and Bao, Y. (2014) Temporal windows as bridge from objective time to subjective time. In D. Lloyd and V. Arstila (Eds.), *Subjective Time: the philosophy, psychology, and neuroscience of temporality*, pp. 241-261, Cambridge: MIT Press.
Pöppel, E. and Harvey, L.O., Jr. (1973) Light-difference threshold and subjective brightness in the periphery of the visual field. *Psychologische Forschung*, *36*,145-161.

Pöppel, E. and Ruhnau, E. (2011) Psychologie als eine auf Modelle angewiesene Angelegenheit ohne Taxonomie – eine Polemik. (Psychology as an enterprise using models without a taxonomy – a polemic). Nova Acta Leopoldina NF 110, Nr. 377, 213-233.

Roenneberg, T. (1996) The complex circadian system of *Gonyaulax polyedra. Physiologica Plantarum* 96, 733-737.

Roenneberg, T. and Pöppel, E. (1985) Topographical distribution of the summation property of Y-ganglion cells in the cat retina. *Experimental Brain Research, 59*, 1-9.

Scoville, W. B. and Milner, B. (1957) Loss of recent memory after bilateral hippocampal lesion. *J. Neuro. Neurosurg. Psych., 20,* 11-21.

Silveira, S., Bao, Y., Wang, L., Pöppel, E., Avram, M., Simmank, F., Zaytseva, Y. and Blautzik, J. (2015) Does a bishop pray when he prays? And does his brain distinguish between different religions? *PsyCh Journal* 4, 199-207. DOI: 10.1002/pchj.116.

Silveira, S., Graupmann, V., Frey, D., Blautzik, J., Meindl, T., Reiser, M., Chen, C., Wang, Y., Bao, Y., Pöppel, E. and Gutyrchik, E. (2012) Matching reality in the arts: Self-referential neural processing of naturalistic compared to surrealistic images. *Perception* 41, 569-576.

Silveira, S., Gutyrchik, E., Wetherell, G., Bao, Y., Pöppel, E., Blautzik, J., Reiser, M., Frey, D. and Graupmann, V. (2014) Ceci n'est pas la mort: Evidence for the recruitment of self-reference from surrealistic art under mortality salience. European Journal of Social Psychology, DOI:10.1002/ejsp.2076.

Sperry, R. (1961) Cerebral organization and behavior. *Science, 133*, 1749-1757.

Stevens, S. S. (1975) *Psychophysics. Introduction to its Perceptual, Neural and Social Prospects.* New York, Wiley.

Vedder, V., Smigielski, L., Gutyrchik, E., Bao, Y., Blautzik, J., Pöppel, E., Zaytseva, Y. and Russell, E. (2015) Neurofunctional Correlates of Environmental Cognition: An fMRI Study with Images from Episodic Memory. *PloS ONE* 10(4): e0122470. doi:10.1371/journal. pone.0122470.

Wang, L., Lin, X., Zhou, B., Pöppel, E. and Bao, Y. (2015) Subjective present: a window of temporal integration indexed by mismatch negativity. *Cognitive Processing*, DOI 10.1007/s10339-015-0687-8.

Wundt, W. (1911) *Einführung in die Psychologie (Introduction into psychology)*. Leipzig: Voigtländer.

Zaytseva, Y., Chan, R. C. K., Pöppel, E. and Heinz, A. (2015) Luria revisited: cognitive research in schizophrenia, past implications and future challenges. *PEHM: Philosophy, Ethics, and Humanities in Medicine* 10:4, DOI10.1186/s13010-015-0026-9.

Zaytseva, Y., Gutyrchik, E., Bao, Y., Pöppel, E., Han, S., Northoff, G., Welker, L., Meindl, T. and Blautzik, J. (2014) Self processing in the brain: A paradigmatic fMRI case study with a professional singer. *Brain and Cognition* 87, 104-108.

Zeki, S., Romaya, J. P., Benincasa, D. M. T. and Atiyah, M. F. (2014) The experience of mathematical beauty and its neural correlates. *Frontiers in Human Neuroscience.* doi.org/10.3389/fnhum.2014.00068.

Zhou, B., Pöppel, E. and Bao, Y. (2014) In the jungle of time: The concept of identity as an escape. *Frontiers in Psychology*, doi: 10.3389/fpsyg.2014.00844.

Zhou, B., Bao, Y., Sander, T., Trahms, L. and Pöppel, E. (2010) Dissociation of summation and peak latencies in visual processing: An MEG study on stimulus eccentricity. *Neuroscience Letters, 483*, 101-104.

Zhou, B., Pöppel, E., Wang, L., Yang, T., Zaytseva, Y. and Bao, Y. (2016) Seeing without knowing: Operational principles along the early visual pathway. *PsyCh Journal*, 5, in press.

Zihl, J., Lissy, P. and Pöppel, E. (1980) Brightness perception in the visual field: Effects of retinal position and adaptation level. *Psychological Research 41*, 297-304.

7 When Brains Design/Experience Buildings: Architectural Patterns for a Good Life

Michael A. Arbib

University of California at San Diego
New School of Architecture and Design, San Diego
arbib@usc.edu

East-West Connections

This chapter is based on a talk presented at a Workshop sponsored by the organization *Para Limes* (Beyond Boundaries) at Nanyang Technological University, Singapore, on September 16, 2015. In my initial planning of a talk that would go "beyond boundaries," I decided to talk on recent efforts to bridge the boundary between thinking about the brain and thinking about buildings, an effort associated with the Academy of Neuroscience for Architecture (www.anfarch.org). But the talk I initially planned did not fully address the title of the Workshop, "East-West Connections: Cultural Patterns, Cognitive Patterns and a Good Life." Let me start then by confronting the challenges posed by this title before I turn to the challenges of developing a neuroscience for architecture to assess what happens when brains design buildings and when brains experience buildings.

What is East? What is West? What East-West connections are we talking about?' When I was a teenager I went to London from Australia and found a Piccadilly Circus where classic London buildings were encrusted in, and transformed by, huge neon signs. And I went to New York which was a totally different kind of city, *the* city of skyscrapers at the middle of the twentieth century. Fast forward to 2000, and we are in the Ginza in Tokyo and we see tall modern buildings totally covered in neon with both Roman and Japanese writing – Piccadilly Circus and New York with Japanese characteristics. Are we in the East, are we in the West? We are in a novel synthesis. Rather than a hard and fast division of East (Japan) and West (UK, US), we see the diffusion of varied notions between East and West.

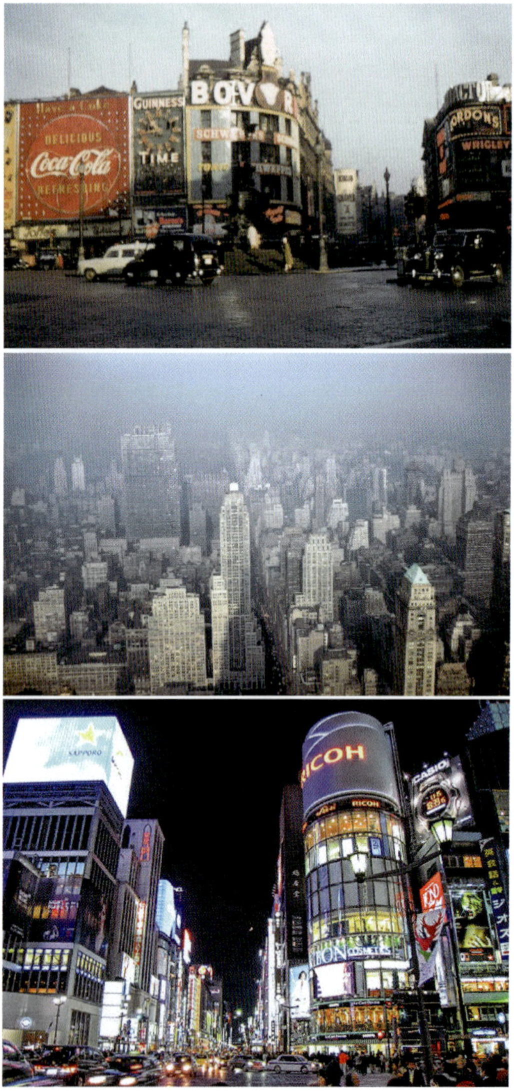

Fig. 1. (Top) Piccadilly Circus, London (1956). (Middle) New York skyscrapers (1956). (Bottom) Ginza, Tokyo (c. 2000).

So what is the East? Is it China, or India, or Japan? But if you talk about Japan, is it the closed Japan before Commodore Perry came? Is it the imperialist colonialist Japan that rampaged over Singapore as well as other places? Is it the modern Japan still informed by the terrible experience of Hiroshima? Or what about China? Imperial China? Maoist

China? Today's China? But where in China? Lhasa or Shanghai? And so on and so on.

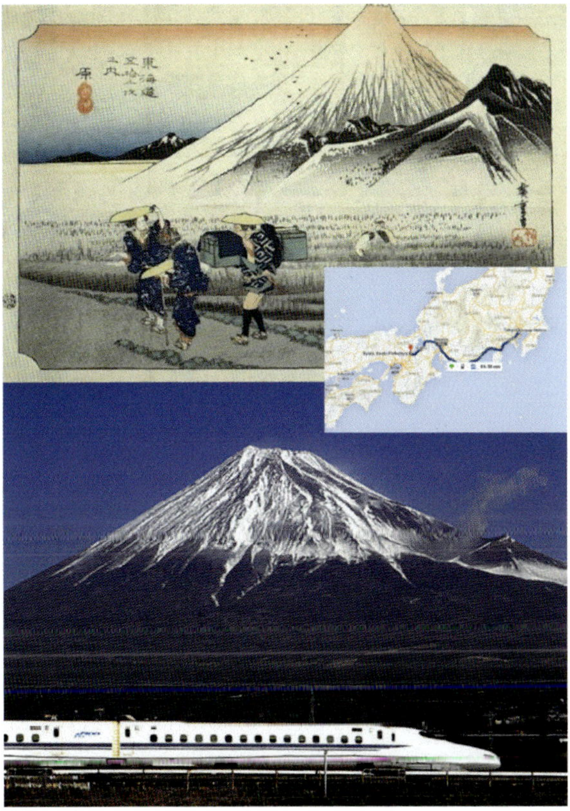

Fig. 2. Fuji, old and new, with an East-West connection.

To illustrate this, Fig. 2 shows two different views of Mt Fuji that make the point that is not just *where* in the East, it is *when* in the East. At the top we see a classic view of Fuji while at the bottom we see this icon of traditional Japan together with the Shinkansen, the modern Japanese elaboration of the British invention, the railway. Appropriately, for the theme of the Workshop, the insert shows that the Shinkansen line from Tokyo to Kyoto that runs past Fuji is indeed an East-West connection!

Similarly, where and when in the West? Historically, we think of Europe as the land of Christendom but what about the Renaissance, or the Enlightenment or Nazism? Thinking of the US as the modern frontier of the West, do you think of it in terms of Liberty and the American Revolution or do you think in terms of slavery? What about colonialism?

We live in a world that even in places that threw off their colonial masters, many (not all) cultural patterns inherited from the former colonial power are admirable. Tellingly, Great Britain was a colonial power but also the source of the Industrial Revolution that gave rise to the modern world.

Such analysis could continue and probe more deeply, but the point that emerges thus far is that East and West are, at least to my mind, not very helpful categories when it comes to assessing the cultural patterns of the modern world, even though the experience of different histories in different regions may shape crucial aspects of modern cultural patterns. We can still fruitfully study what makes different parts of the *geographical* East (Asia, perhaps) different from each other and from different parts of the West, yet learn too from the historical processes of cross-fertilization between them.

A Good Life

The other challenge posed by the Workshop title is to assess what defines a good life. But this topic is so vast that I will simply catalogue a few aspects of relevance to this chapter.

Obvious factors are to have a good place to live, a good job, a happy family. Yet is a life in which you have a job and you work 9 to 5 and you go home and watch television and eat noodles and the same thing happens day after day really a good life? It is a comfortable life. Many aspects of physical well-being are certainly taken care of. But surely more is required to live a truly good life? A life without beauty or without surmounting individual challenge seems somehow not to be a truly good life.

For others, comfort and beauty do not suffice without the experience of individual freedom – but what is experienced as freedom depends very much on cultural pattern. Is it freedom to do whatever you want to? I think that freedom without constraints is not freedom; it must be yoked to some notion of purpose. But is your sense of purpose to be defined with respect to some intellectual goals? Or with respect to some pride in your nation and being a contributor to the nation? Or perhaps it is rooted in a religious framework in which a good life is not one that makes you feel good now but rather one that prepares you for eternal heavenly bliss, or a good reincarnation or, again, in terms of any other of many cultural patterns.

Pondering the themes of this meeting got me to restructure my thinking about the linkage between neuroscience and architecture, leading me to assess to what extent we can view architecture as the attempt to design and build buildings and spaces that support a good life. For those who judge architecture mainly on the basis of pictures in glossy magazines, perhaps beauty in some sense of aesthetic judgement is all that matters. But what about the need for homes that supports the well-being of a family? And the architecture of public buildings and spaces may be judged in terms of a sense of community as another ingredient of a good life. In fact, most of us are part of multiple communities, even strange communities that gather to talk about the good life in Singapore from time to time.

So public spaces create a sense of community and we need public institutions to support a good life: good systems of law, good systems of education and so on. For each of these, extensive and conflicting tomes have been written on what constitutes a "good" or "fair" or "just" system, but here (briefly) our focus is on the extent to which architecture can provide buildings that not only are effective in supporting the services that these functions demand but can also create symbolic forms that give citizens the feeling that they are parts of this well-established structure. There are also buildings, prisons for example, where the inmates are not offered a sense of belonging but those outside may be offered a sense of the workings of the law. With this I turn to my first example of public institutions, namely sacred spaces, and here I will start with an explicit contrast between East and West.

Sacred Spaces

Figure 3 shows the exterior and interior of the Todai-ji temple in Nara in Japan, and the cathedral of Notre Dame in Paris. As you enter Todai-Ji, two huge Buddhas tower above you. The photographer used an exposure of 1/30 sec to bring up detail from the shadows (Bartel, 2013) whereas when you enter the temple you come into a dark space – but your eyes are lifted up to see the faces of these Buddhas and somehow that contemplation with raised gaze is part of your religious experience. We can contrast that with that icon of Christian architecture – Notre Dame in Paris. Here the light, rather than being excluded as our eyes rise up, is everywhere, as exemplified by the rose window.

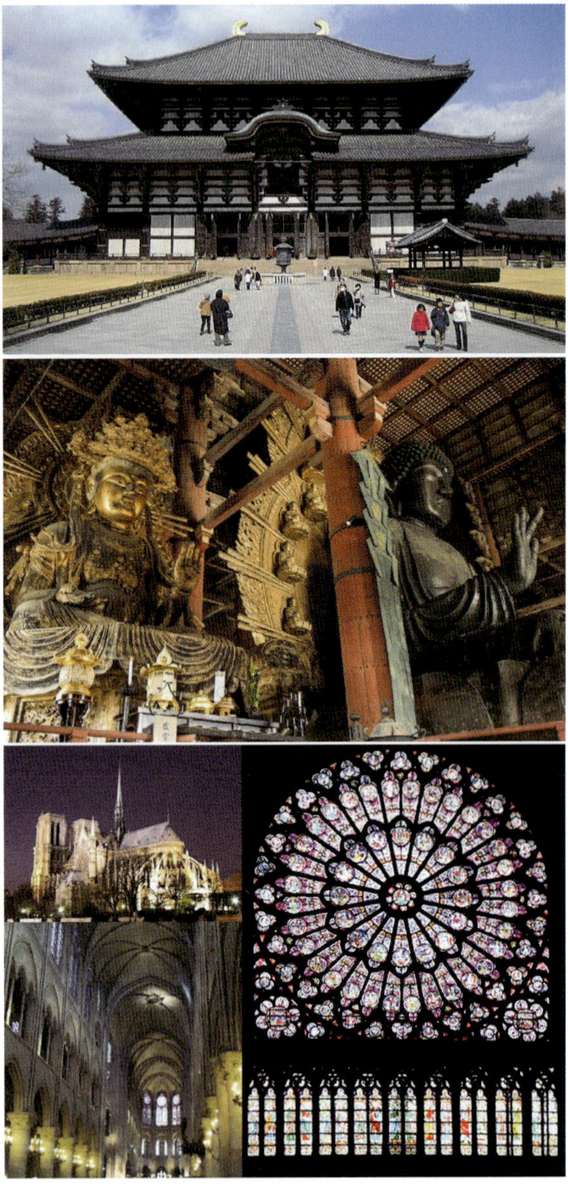

Fig. 3. Sacred spaces in East (Japan, Buddhism) and West (France, Christianity). (Top and middle) Todai-Ji in Nara. (Bottom) Notre Dame in Paris.

Cultural patterns are crucial here – a Buddhist will have a far deeper experience at Todai-Ji than will a Christian, and vice versa in Notre Dame. In one case, the huge figures of the Buddha hold deep meaning;

in the other a much smaller statue of a person being tortured to death on two pieces of wood signifies the grace of God. A dramatic cultural contrast. If you keep looking around you in a Christian church, you may see beautiful statues of the Madonna; and if you explore Nara, you will see fearsome guardian angels. A scholar of comparative religion may then descry deep commonalities among the cultural contrasts, but here I want to focus on one *architectural* commonality between these sacred spaces – raising the eyes up from the earthly plane towards something that is beyond our everyday experience.

I want to stress that the raising of the gaze – the experience within the building – cannot be captured in a visual image, though different images may serve different purposes (Neutra, 2014). Rather, a crucial aspect of a building is how one interacts with it, whether in exploring it, or in putting it to use in quotidian tasks or in activities of deep significance. Moreover, one's interactions may include senses beyond the visual: the sound of footsteps, the wafting of incense, the singing of the choir may all augment one's experience of a religious ceremony in Notre Dame.

Having said all this, though, one of the first attempts to explore the neural correlates of experiencing sacred spaces used photographs to elicit subjects' responses. Bermudez, Krizaj, Lipschitz, Debborah, and Nakamura (2014) used fMRI (functional magnetic resonance imaging). The general methodology is to have subjects perform two different tasks (possibly many times, using variations of the task to gain statistical power) and the brain is scanned each time. Powerful magnetic fields, arrays of sensors, and massive computing combine to locate regions where blood flow is significantly greater in one task than the other. I have suggested that we need a "vampire model" of the neuron to link the blood flow in a region (how much blood the neurons there "suck" to support their metabolism) to the activity of neurons in the region, so that we can test hypotheses about what computations at the neural level might underlie the task-dependent differences seen in the fMRI. The smallest volume element in an fMRI image represents the time- and space-smeared activity of millions of neurons. But what aspect of the activity of individual neurons is contributing to signal in the image? It seems to depend more on the degree of synaptic activity (the push and pull between excitation and inhibition) than on the actual firing rate of neurons (Arbib *et al.*, 2000; Bonaiuto and Arbib, 2014).

For Bermudez and his colleagues, the two tasks were to look at pictures of (A) "ordinary" buildings versus (B) "contemplation-inducing" buildings. They found some overlap of regions more active for task B with regions other studies had found to be active during contemplation (Cahn and Polich, 2006). They interviewed the subjects after the scanning and found correlations between subject-reported anxiety, depth of experience and brain physiology attributable to the induced contemplation. This is a pioneering attempt but is limited in ways which we must assess in charting further directions in neuroscience for architecture.

First, subjects were experiencing pictures rather than the space around and within actual buildings. We cannot carry out fMRI studies of people moving around buildings though we can get "halfway there" by exploiting virtual reality. Another methodology is to use electroencephalography (EEG) which exchanges the relatively precise localization of brain activity of fMRI for more precise timing – and EEG can be recorded with portable "helmets" rather than large, immovable multi-million dollar machines. So the challenge remains of getting comparable data when people are actually in Todai-Ji or Notre Dame.

Second is the challenge of more fully characterizing what subjects are reacting to. If I see a building, I may recognize that it is a holy space, a relatively "cold" reaction compared to the lived multisensory experience of the sounds of the choir reflected by the soaring ceiling, the light streaming through the rose window, and more, and this experience may differ in turn to the extent to which I am steeped in the cultural patterns of the religion for which the building was constructed.

The third challenge, then, is the need to tease apart the neural correlates of different cultural patterns – e.g., to tease apart the experiences of Todai-Ji for a Southern Baptist and a devout Buddhist. Much work has to be done to better understand the neuro-correlations of sacred space, and the challenges only multiply when we turn to other types of buildings.

Neuroscience and Cognitive Science and the Understanding of the Processes of Architecture

In a classic study of psychological and medical effects of architectural choices, Ulrich (1984) studied recovery after the same surgery of 46 patients in a suburban Pennsylvania hospital between 1972 and 1981. The 23 patients assigned to rooms with windows looking out on a natural scene had shorter postoperative hospital stays and took fewer painkillers than 23 matched patients in similar rooms with windows facing a brick building wall. This provides hard data for what is perhaps the commonsense view that engagement with nature is part of a good life – and here the way it enhances human well-being could be measured within the context of hospital design. Is it enough to build a better architecture for a good life to learn from behavioral data or can more be gained by knowing what's going on in people's brains? I think the jury is still out, but I am going to show you pathways of connection, crossing the boundaries (para limes) between neuroscience and architecture.

But first I need to discuss what neuroscience is and is not. Consider the triad of experience, behavior and brain. If we think about architecture purely in terms of beautiful pictures in the glossy magazines, or the brief glimpse of a building by a tourist just passing by, then we might frame everything in terms of visual experience. But if it is a building that we actually use, whether to pray or to fill in forms or to go to school or live in as a home, then our behavior is crucial. What counts is not just the visual experience as a mere observer, it is the linkage of experience and behavior of somebody using the building, somebody acting, interacting. When we seek to link the study of that behavior and experience to analysis of possible underlying "computations," we are engaged in *cognitive science*.

If we try to go further and re-characterize those computations in such a way that we understand how different parts of the brain contribute to them, then we move on to *cognitive neuroscience* – studying brain, behavior and experience in an integrated way. Juhani Pallasmaa, the dean of Finnish architects and the author of many excellent books that stress the multisensory nature of the experience of architecture (Pallasmaa, 2009, 2012), developed a phenomenology of architecture: understanding architecture in terms of the way we experience it – see his chapter in *Mind in Architecture: Neuroscience, Embodiment, and the Future of Design* (Robinson and Pallasmaa, 2015). Neuroscience enriches this phenomenology, illuminating it by showing how, as a person's brain changes or for people with different brains, then what they experience is different. Therefore, having an understanding of different brain types and how that affects perception and action will enrich the phenomenology of knowing how different people experience different buildings. Having said that, I would add that the study of behavior and experience in phenomenological and cognitive terms forms a necessary complement to "pure" neuroscience in the development of a neuroscience for architecture that is the aim for ANFA – one cannot jump directly from the reality of lived experience to the dynamics of neural

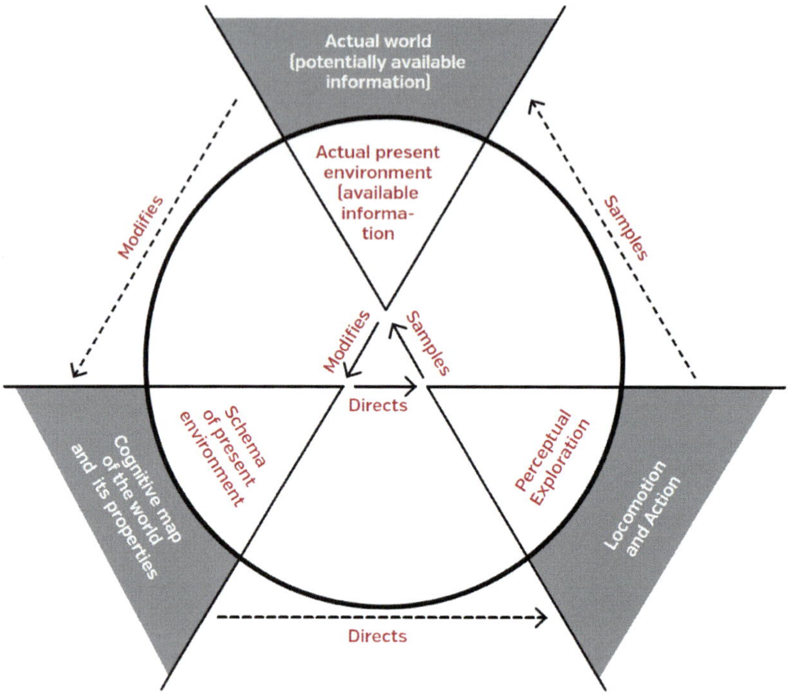

Fig. 4. The action-perception cycle (adapted from Neisser, 1976).

networks without the consideration of mediating levels of representation (Arbib, 2013a).

I want to reiterate that we are not just concerned with passive perceptual experience. We need to understand how we experience the world as we interact with it. Figure 4 is based on Ulric Neisser's (Neisser, 1976) notion of what I call the Action-Perception Cycle (Arbib, 1989). The key idea is that at any particular time what we perceive is not a neutral stimulus but depends in great part on our then current needs and goals and motivations. Indeed, some of our behaviors are efforts to explore the environment seeking information relevant to our current tasks – and this will inform our praxic and social actions, our physical task-oriented actions in the world and our social interactions. As we act, new sensory data flow in to be interpreted in terms of our current goals and ideas, possibly changing them in the process.

The action-perception cycle is a learning cycle, too, because as we interact with the world our new experiences, especially those that are unexpected or otherwise memorable, change our brains and thus alter the dynamics of the cycle as we continue to confront new situations. Famously, the pre-Socratic Greek philosopher Heraclitus (535-475 BC) said *"you can never step in the same river twice."* As a neuroscientist, I would say "*you can never think with the same brain twice*."

To continue with this emphasis on an action-oriented view of perception, we turn to the notion of an *affordance* (Gibson, 1966, 1979). A motivating example for J.J. Gibson was that of a pilot landing a plane: it is not necessary for him to identify all the objects at the airfield; rather it is the pattern of optic flow from the runway, the way that pattern from the environment creates flow of activity across the retina, that provides the crucial information needed to decide (subconsciously, if he is a skilled pilot) at what rate to descend, when to level out, and so on.

Imagine that you are walking down La Rambla in Barcelona and that you are looking at various sights along the way, but suddenly you swerve. Why did you do that? Because your peripheral vision picked up the imminence of a possible collision and subconsciously your brain directed you to avoid that collision. This requires no conscious attention to what caused you to swerve – and if that "obstacle" was a friend of yours, you might receive an aggrieved phone call asking why you snubbed them. Turvey and his colleagues (Turvey, 1992; Turvey and Shaw, 1978) introduced the dual notion of *effectivity* – the motor capabilities for action that complement the perceptual detection of affordances for action. Indeed, my colleagues and I have exploited human behavioral studies of humans, neurophysiological studies of monkeys, and computational modeling to explore the neural mechanisms underlying the role of affordances in visual control of reaching and grasping (Fagg and Arbib, 1998; Jeannerod *et al.*, 1995). Elsewhere (Arbib, 2015), I have briefly considered the relevance of such studies to the issues raised by Juhani Pallasmaa for architecture in *The Thinking Hand* (Pallasmaa, 2009).

Three Ways to Link Architecture and Neuroscience

This is where the story of the interaction between architecture and neuroscience really starts. I have divided it into three facets:

The one most addressed within ANFA is *the neuroscience of the experience of architecture*. We seek to understand what is going through somebody's head as they occupy a room, or behave in the context of different buildings. This is tightly connected with the second facet, *the neuroscience of the design process*, assessing what is going on in the head of the architect as he or she tries to envision the experience of inhabitants and design the building according to some criteria for what constitutes a good experience, both aesthetically and functionally. The third facet is *neuromorphic architecture*, assessing what it would mean for a building to "have a brain." In this section, I will briefly discuss the neuroscience of the experience of architecture and neuromorphic architecture and will turn later to the neuroscience of the design process.

The neuroscience of the experience of architecture was well defined by John Paul Eberhard, who was the founding president of ANFA. In his book *Brain Landscape: The Coexistence of Neuroscience and Architecture* (Eberhard, 2008) he stressed that buildings where people spend much time can influence the fundamental structure of the brain and thus affect people's thoughts and behaviors. His goal was to foster development of a "database" of neuroscience results that have important implications for understanding how different populations will experience and benefit from schools, homes for Alzheimer's patients, diverse workplaces, sacred spaces, and more. The good life is not a universal: one must ask for Whom? When? Where? Understanding the neural underpinnings of memory loss can inform the design of residences for Alzheimer's patients (Zeisel, 2006); understanding the neuroplasticity of young brains can help us understand what makes an effective learning environment, and so on. Alas, the database envisaged by Eberhard does not yet exist, but steps towards its creation can be seen by reading the abstracts and viewing the videos of presentations at the ANFA Conferences held in 2012 and 2014:

http://www.anfarch.org/2012-anfa-conference/,
http://www.anfarch.org/2014-conference/.

In each case mentioned above, we are dealing with people with very different brains, the brains of the young, the alas badly memory-impaired brains of some of the old, and the brains of people in their prime engaged in different specialized activities. But one of the things that really hit me as I reconsidered the conversation between architecture and neuroscience while assessing the nature of "a good life" was the importance of politics. For example, if we talk about a good life in the workplace, then whose is the good life? Is it the good life of the type of owner who maximizes productivity as a means to greater profits or the good life of the worker who gets to enjoy his work and gets a decent salary? One may hope that the person commissioning the design of the workplace would take full account of the needs of the workers in balancing the two, but the architecture of the building would be very different depending on which answers are made to such political questions. Further consideration of this lies outside the scope of this article, but it does show the challenge of *Para Limes* – the way in which our attempt to move beyond one boundary may lead us to cross other boundaries as well, leading us into territory for which our own expertise leaves us ill-prepared, compounding the current challenge of enriching the cross-border traffic between architecture and neuroscience.

With this we turn to neuromorphic architecture, the idea of "brains" for buildings. Much of my neuroscience work contributed to the field of computational neuroethology (Cliff, 2002) – developing computational models of the neural mechanisms relevant to ethology (the study of animal behavior) – be the animals frogs, monkeys, rats ... or humans (Arbib, 2003). How do animals interact with the world around them, whether in the physical or social world? We study an agent looking out at the world, and seek to understand what it is about the brain that supports these interactions with the world out there. Almost every year from 1986 to 2015 I gave a course on "Brain Theory and Artificial Intelligence" at USC, the University of Southern California. In 2003 and 2004, I asked students to conduct projects that developed "Brains for Intelligent Rooms." We turned neuroethology inside out – instead of an animal in its environment, we considered "intelligent" rooms that surrounded their environment. Such a room's sensors are directed inwards. In today's surveillance society such an idea is common; the issue then was to investigate what the study of neuroscience can add to the "information infrastructure" of a room or building so that it could better serve its inhabitants (rather than serving those who choose to monitor them – politics again). I am not going to pursue this topic further here (see Arbib, 2012, for more on "Brains, Machines, and Buildings") but I do want to present (Fig. 5) the poster for a talk I gave a few years ago since its visual pun also introduces the notion of eco-architecture to which we return later in the paper.

ANFA INTERFACES

A series of discussions about emerging research at the intersection of
Neuroscience and Architecture

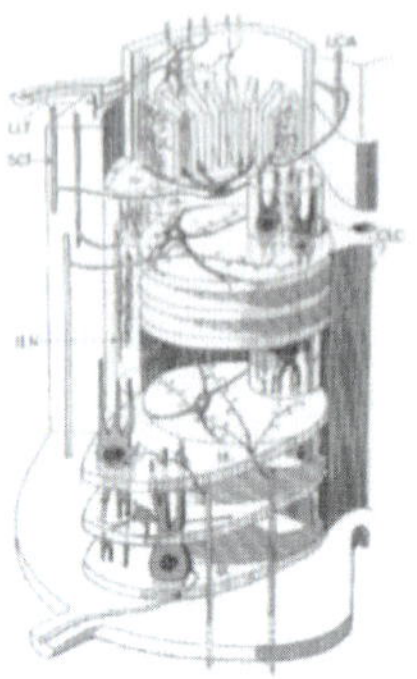

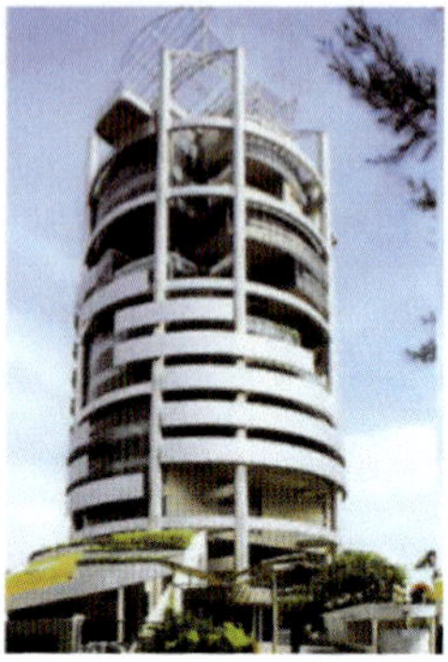

Brains, Machines and Buildings

Fig. 5. (Left) John Szentágothai's drawing of the neuroanatomy of the spinal cord. (Right) Ken Yeang's (1992) IBM Tower, Kuala Lumpur.

On the left is a diagram by Janos Szentágothai, Hungary's greatest neuroanatomist, that indicates the three-dimensional arrangement of neurons within the spinal cord (adapted from Szentágothai and Réthelyi, 1973). When the architect Ben Arbib saw this he recognized the striking visual similarity to Ken Yeang's 1992 IBM Tower (across the water from Singapore in Kuala Lumpur), shown at right. There is no relation between the neuroanatomy at left and the architecture at right – there is just a fascinating visual coincidence between the two pictures. But the reason it is worth attending to Fig. 5 (now that we leave the theme of neuromorphic architecture) is that Ken Yeang was a pioneer of *eco-architecture* (Hart, 2011), the design of buildings in an ecological way. A strategy to reduce the energy consumption exemplified here is to bring greenery into the building, and to design open spaces that can exploit natural breezes to reduce, or avoid, the need for air-conditioning – bringing techniques that may be thousands of years old in tropical countries into modern architecture.

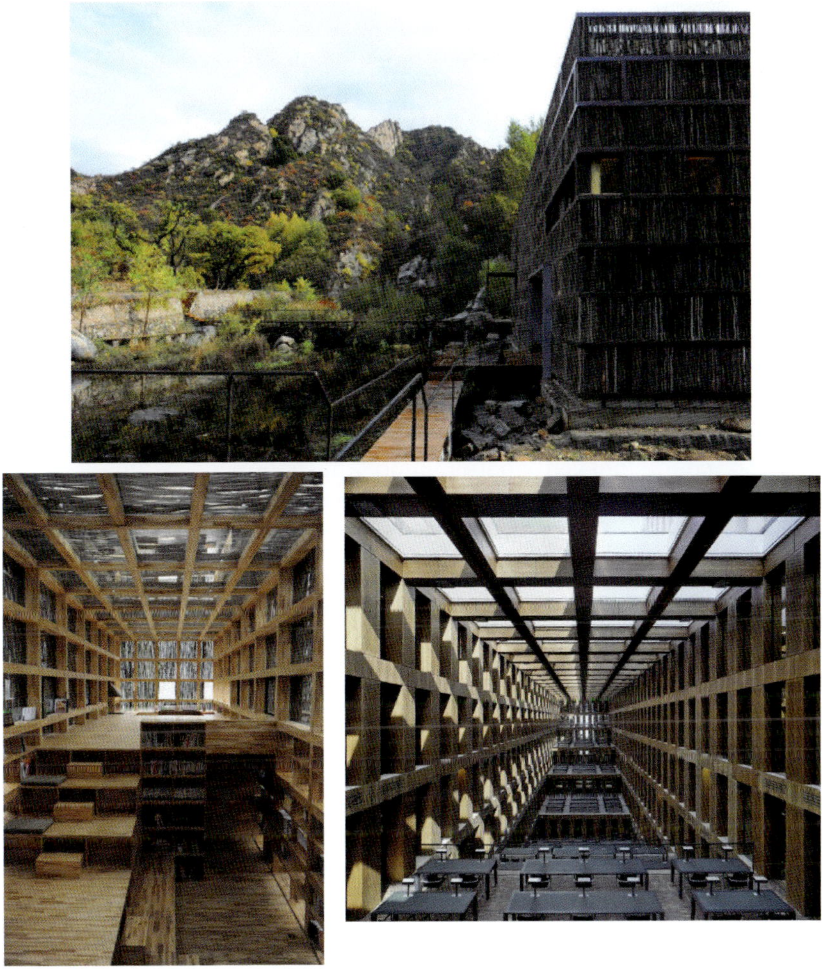

Fig. 6. (Top) A small library with Chinese characteristics. (Bottom left) An interior view. (Bottom right) A strikingly similar interior for a large library.

We thus see eco-architecture not only as an important approach to building a good life through architecture, but also as evidence of *the interplay of cultural patterns and geographical realities* – an eco-architecture for the tropics would have little value in Sweden, for example, where heavy winters must be dealt with. Here we see a cultural pattern that is not an arbitrary accident of history but as something that reflects the adaptation of a set of design principles to conditions in a particular region of the world. All this suggests the value for architecture of a conversation between traditional technology and modern technology to yield new syntheses, new cultural patterns rooted in the old and yet informed by the diversity of patterns emerging in the multiple cultures of East and West.

Figure 6 shows a small library "with Chinese characteristics," the LiYuan Library of 2011, designed by Li Xiaodong Atelier and situated a couple of hours outside Beijing. It is a modern library and yet one has the sense that feel for both the Chinese countryside and for Chinese cultural patterns went into the design of this library. But consider now the library shown at bottom right in Fig. 6. The resemblance between the two interiors is striking – and yet the second library is not in China, but is the library of the Jacob and Wilhelm Grimm Centre of 2009 in Berlin, architect Max Dudler. We see here a striking convergence, where what seemed at first (given the sequencing of this article) a design with Chinese characteristics shares important geometric features with a modern Western design. This is just to say that there are both distinctive cultural patterns and there are international commonalities, whether through explicit sharing or happy coincidence.

Libraries

With this, let me further consider libraries as a key example of buildings that provide a community with an institution for a good life on a social scale. This section builds on the presentations at a session "Science + Form = Function: The Impact of Neuroscience on Architecture & Design" at the annual meeting of the American Library Association (ALA) in June 2014 in Las Vegas. It was organized by Eric Kidwell of the Houghton Memorial Library of Huntingdon College in Alabama and the speakers were Ken Kornberg, an architect from the Bay area of San Francisco and a member of the ANFA Board of Directors (Kornberg, 2014), Hannah Bennett, who was then the architecture librarian at Princeton University (Bennett, 2013, 2014), and myself.

Traditionally, the library was a place to go to get books and reading material. From 1883 to 1929, 1,689 Carnegie Libraries were built in the United States, playing a vital role in small towns, providing people access to the world of literature, diversion, and knowledge. Today, the library is perhaps less relevant when people can log onto the Web to satisfy these needs. In fact, when I talk to some librarians and architects, they say that not only has the downgrading of books in favor of access to digital media changed the face of library design but that a major design consideration for urban libraries is now the care of the homeless who find it a place of refuge from the street. But in the rest of this section I am going to focus on libraries in a more traditional sense.

Library functions	**Experiencing architecture**
•Data collection	•Vision: shape, color, order ...
•Storage: stacks, archives	•Smell: flowers, books, wood ...
•Presentation: art, books, & more	•Taste: coffee plus
•Reading	•Sound: quiet, loud, distracting ...
•Contemplation	•Touch: texture
•Meeting, conference	•Pressure: heights, humidity, HVAC
•Studying	•Balance: floors, patterns, stairs, levels
•Teaching	•Temperature: comfort, attraction
•Refuge	•Pain: emotional, physical
	•Motion: time, space

Fig. 7. Library functions and sensory experience (adapted from a slide of Ken Kornberg at the ALA meeting, June 2014).

Figure 7 is based on the ALA talk by Ken Kornberg. The left-hand column reminds us of the diversity of functions a library may serve: collecting data and storing it; presenting it for people to read or contemplate, and much more. The relative balance of the different functions can radically affect the design of the library: Is access to books the key? Or is it a place to use the Internet while talking to people searching for similar information? The right-hand column shows diverse contributions the different senses make to experiencing architecture. In the spirit of the action-perception cycle (Fig. 4), we can note the different ways these systems come into play as we engage in actions serving the different functions listed at left. The taste of the coffee in the lounge; the sound – is it quiet, loud, or distracting?; the texture of the books and tables; and the encounters as we and others move through the space to find books and media and interact with them. All this reminds us of the importance of the melding of action and perception by the embodied user, taking us beyond the mere surfaces of visual appearance (important though they may be in setting an aesthetic framework for our experiences as we go about our tasks in the building). The right-hand column gives us a small sample of diverse sensory systems, and each of these engage a different specialty in neuroscience. Will the details of the brain's workings inform tomorrow's architecture? Just as today no architect would complete the design of a building without consulting a structural engineer, the day may come when large architectural projects will benefit from consultation with a neuro-engineer. But that day has not yet arrived.

In her ALA talk, Hannah Bennett analyzed the architecture of libraries in a very different way, stressing symbolic value. For example, one approaches Gunnar Asplund's Stockholm City Library by an impressive walkway that leads up to the entrance and then one ascends a yet more impressive staircase before you finally reach the reading room, a massive cylindrical structure whose lower walls are covered by tier upon tier of books. This approach symbolizes the ascent to knowledge and is designed to inculcate a reverence for learning as you ascend towards the space where the books are so displayed as to impress you with the breadth of knowledge that they contain. (Campbell and Pryce (2013) presented a world history with fine photographs and discussions of libraries from around the world and up to the present day, including Asplund's library on pp.254-260.)

To pursue this theme, consider the Doheny Memorial Library at the University of Southern California (Fig. 8). One ascends stairs to enter the building, and then ascends a further flight of stairs, looking up to the Great Hall as one does so. Ruth Wallach, formerly the architecture librarian at USC (Fig. 8 assembles four of her photos) comments that the Great Hall is "symbolic of the realm of wisdom and truth." But as one passes through the brightly-lit door to enter the stacks, she is no longer impressed: "An unprepossessing entryway, a narrow door into a compressed space, the stacks. One feels like an animal burrowing underground. No natural light, compressed space, low ceilings." Not good – but let us be fair to the architect. This library was built in the days when the stacks were closed, so only the librarians had to suffer these compressed spaces. The architects' only design criterion was to get as many books as possible into the stacks and still make them accessible. But Ben Arbib had a different view of the stacks when he was a student at USC, speaking of the "low ceiling, isolated desks in nooks and crannies; the drum of the air conditioning. Being lost and finding yourself. Finding unexpected books as you scan the stacks." For him, it was not the aesthetic or symbolic value of the library that mattered. It was not ease of the wayfinding we will discuss in the next section. It was the joy of exploration.

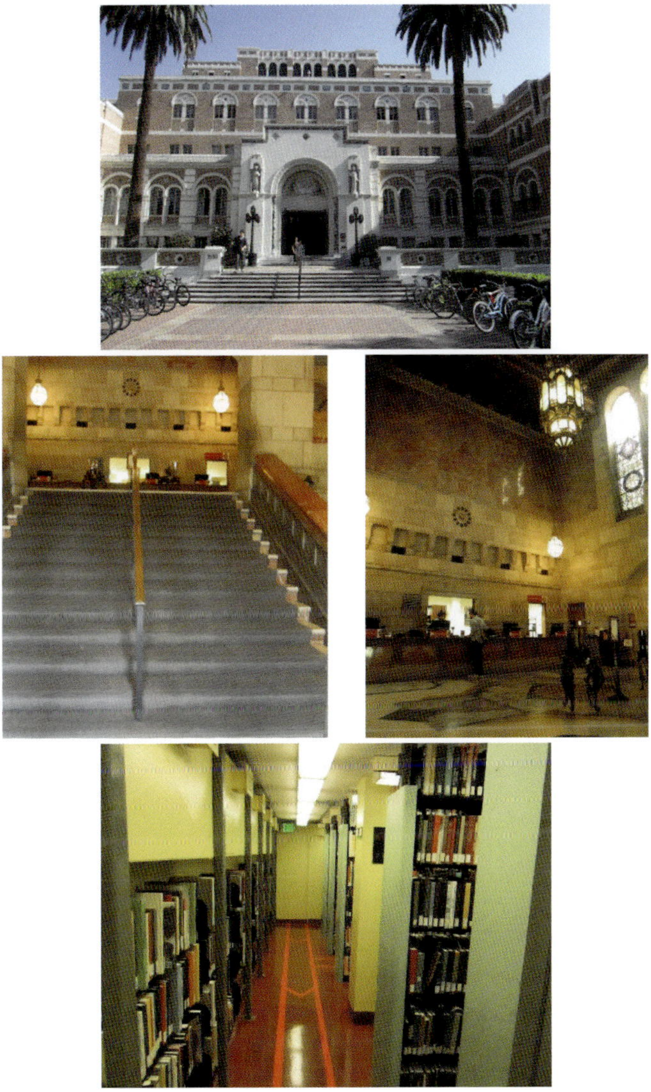

Fig. 8. The Doheny Memorial Library at the University of Southern California. (Top) Exterior view. (Middle) After entering the doors, one ascends the staircase to reach the Great Hall. (Bottom) On entering the stacks, the symbolic values of the Great Hall are left behind. (Photographs courtesy of Ruth Wallach.)

And so here is another politico-architectural consideration. When you think about society, do you want a regimented society with responsibilities and rewards all laid out for you? Or do you want an expansive society where the possibility of failure may be balanced by the excitement of finding your own path to success? Similar questions may apply to architecture and urban design (or organic growth). Venice is one of my favorite cities precisely because I can get lost there. I come out on the edge of a canal and see the bridge I seek off to my right. I explore various alleyways to return to the canal – and there is the bridge to my left. But I am happy rather than frustrated because the buildings are beautiful and the process of exploration is part of what makes a visit to Venice worthwhile even if there is a particular church or a particular theatre that I wish to get to and my arrival is delayed.

Thus as we turn to the question of how to design buildings to help inhabitants find their way, and as we marshal neural data relevant to wayfinding, we must also keep in mind the further challenge (not developed here) of understanding how these same neural systems support exploration, and what motivational systems may govern the tradeoff between finding a path that leads to a place that will satisfy one's immediate needs and exploration that has no immediate payoff but which is motivating in itself and may (or may not) contribute to the knowledge base that will support later wayfinding (Arbib and Bonaiuto, 2012; Lieblich and Arbib, 1982).

Wayfinding

When you come to a new area, how do you find your way? There can be signs, and there can be architectural nudges, such as the relation between stairs, elevators and restrooms. Let us look briefly at Rem Koolhaas's Seattle Public Library (Fig. 9). It has an unusual arrangement in that the stacks are arranged in a spiral with no separate floors or areas, one just traverses up or down the spiral to find what one is looking for. A group in America and Germany looked at this as part of a more general study of wayfinding, offering a cognitive science analysis of why people get lost in buildings (Carlson *et al.*, 2010). Good signage can help alleviate the problem, and another solution would be to make the layout of the building available on a smartphone app and let the app guide people to where they want to go. But the fact remains that the way for example, the architect designs corridors, the way that rooms are distributed, and available lines of sight can all make a building easier or harder to navigate. (How to support the joy of exploration discussed earlier is a different sort of challenge.) Carlson *et al.* showed that Koolhaas's library was in fact a very hard place for people to navigate in.

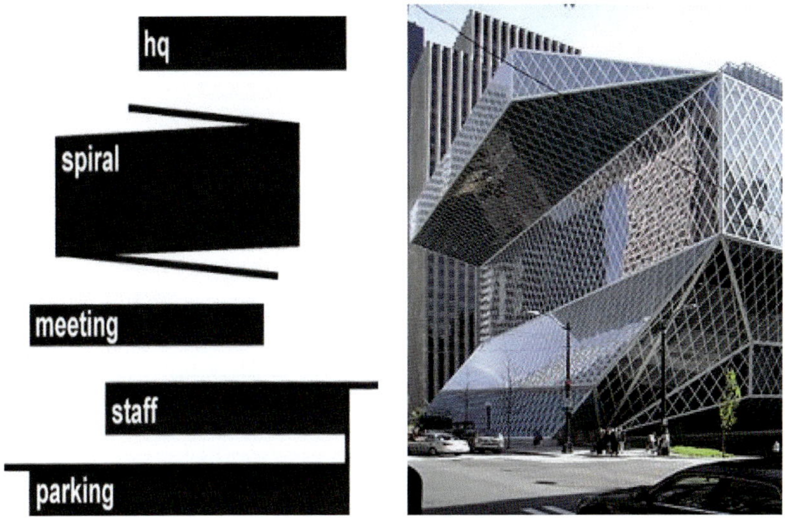

Fig. 9. Layout and exterior view of the Seattle Public Library.

Ken Kornberg, whom we met earlier, designs research buildings including those of the Okinawa Institute of Science and Technology. He likes to use curved corridors because in a big building with long straight corridors one may lose one's sense of direction, but a curved corridor offers the cue of whether the inner curve is on the left or right, which also provides an extra cue as to where a room is located. Neither the practical experience of Kornberg nor the study of Carlson *et al.* link directly to neuroscience but each offers insights into how the analysis of people finding their way in buildings may yield practical advice for architecture.

Let me now bring the neuroscience that comes closest to wayfinding into this mix of behavioral tricks and cognitive studies. The story starts with the discovery of *place cells* by John O'Keefe, neurons in the rat hippocampus whose firing correlated not so much with what the rat perceived or how the rat acted or with what the rat remembered, but rather with the *place* it occupied in the maze in which the experimenter had placed it (O'Keefe and Dostrovsky, 1971). This finding initiated work over the ensuing decades that in 2014 culminated in the award of the Nobel Prize in Physiology or Medicine to John O'Keefe and two other researchers (O'Keefe, 2014). By contrast, the classic study of the hippocampus in the *human* brain comes from study of H.M., a man who had had such bad epilepsy that his surgeon cut out a huge region of his brain, including hippocampus to block the seizures (Scoville and Milner, 1957). Intriguingly for us, but unfortunately for him, H.M. lost the ability to form *episodic memories*, memories of particular episodes he had experienced. He could remember events that had occurred before the operation, but he could not remember subsequent episodes. Yet his working *memory*, his memory of what was of relevance in the current activity of the action-perception cycle, was fine. Nonetheless, once the current dynamics is disrupted, the working memory is lost and no new episodic memory will have been formed. One colleague of mine was conducting a study with him and had what appeared to be a normal conversation, but was called to the phone (back in the old days when one actually had to go to the phone rather than pull it from one's pocket). And when he came back, he apologized to H.M. – but no apology was necessary because H.M. had forgotten that they had met before, let alone been conversing a few minutes earlier.

But researchers had a surprise in store. If they showed H.M., let us say, a new board game he had never seen before, his working memory sufficed for him to follow the exposition of the rules and play the game. But next day, he had no recollection of having seen the game before, and needed to have it explained again. But here was the surprise: as the days went by and he played the game again and again, he became more skillful. Other parts of his brain not involving the hippocampus (which he had lost) were able to build up the synapses to support this new skill. We say that although he lacked episodic memory, he still had *procedural memory* (Squire and Wixted, 2011).

We might call episodic memory the key to wayfinding in times past. Two studies from 2006 by Eleanor Maguire and her colleagues connect the human hippocampus to navigation, to wayfinding in space, and thus offer a bridge back to the detailed study of neural circuits in the rat brain.

Maguire *et al.* (2006), noting the remarkable knowledge of licensed London taxi drivers of all the streets and navigational strategies for the city, compared the taxi drivers with London bus drivers, who were matched for driving experience and levels of stress – but differed in that bus drivers follow a constrained set of routes. Years of navigation experience were found to correlate with hippocampal gray matter volume only in taxi drivers, with right posterior gray matter volume increasing and anterior volume decreasing with more navigation experience. However, the ability to acquire new visuo-spatial information was worse in taxi drivers than in bus drivers. Maguire *et al.* speculated that a complex spatial representation, which facilitates expert navigation and is associated with greater posterior hippocampal gray matter volume, might come at a cost to new spatial memories and gray matter volume in the anterior hippocampus.

In a related study, Maguire *et al.* (2006) used a highly accurate and interactive virtual reality simulation of central London to assess the navigation ability of a licensed London taxi driver (referred to as TT) who had sustained bilateral hippocampal damage. In this test, TT and matched control taxi drivers drove a virtual London taxi along the streets they had first learned 40 years before. Maguire *et al.* found that the hippocampus is not required for general orientation in the city or for detailed topographical knowledge of landmarks and their spatial relationships. However, while TT could navigate reliably on main artery roads, he became lost when navigation depended instead on other roads. Perhaps this is because frequently used routes are multiply represented in hippocampus in ways which make them more resistant to hippocampal damage than infrequently used, and thus perhaps sparsely represented, routes. This still leaves open the issue of the extent to which navigation is carried out within the hippocampus or within a larger system of which hippocampus is just a part (Guazzelli *et al.*, 1998; O'Keefe, 1983).

While the above does not close the gap between the cognitive study of "getting lost in buildings" and neuroscience, it does offer clues as to how the rapprochement might be effected; and the use of interactive virtual reality by Maguire *et al.* (2006) offers an important methodology for carrying out experiments relevant to further development of a neuroscience for architecture. For a step in this direction, see Lelin *et al.* (2010).

Neuroscience of the Design Process

An earlier section briefly discussed *neuromorphic architecture* and the *neuroscience of the experience of architecture*. In this section, we offer a perspective on the *neuroscience of the design process* by briefly assessing what the noted Swiss architect Peter Zumthor had to say in his essay "A Way of Looking At Things" (Zumthor, 2012). (I discuss this topic in more detail in Arbib, 2013b, where I also use an example from choreography to examine group creativity in the development of form in the four dimensions of space and time.) My general hypothesis is that this assessment exemplifies ways in which looking at the processes in the mind of the architect during design may offer interesting challenges for developing new chapters in cognitive neuroscience.

> When I think about architecture, images coming into my mind.
>
> When I design, I frequently find myself sinking into old, half-forgotten memories. ... Yet at the same time, I know that all is new and that there is no direct reference to a former work of architecture.

First note that the "images" here need not be purely visual – as in episodic memory, they may combine action and a range of associated perceptual experience. Earlier we studied H.M. who could not form new episodic memories. Here we have a different perspective in which the aim is *not* to recall past episodes accurately, but rather to recall fragments of such experiences in the service of imagination, of creating new experiences. Thus, factoring what we know about episodic memory into developing the neuroscience of imagination is one of the challenges that will help us bridge the borders between architecture and neuroscience.

> Unlike the sculptor, I have to start with functional and technical requirements.

For a building to be successful it must not just look good, it must be useful.

> The challenge of developing a whole out of innumerable details, out of various functions and forms, materials and dimensions.
>
> Details ... lead to an understanding of the whole of which they are an intrinsic part.

Here the interplay between whole and parts is crucial. A related challenge in analyzing visual perception has been only partly addressed by neuroscience: When I look at a scene, I immediately get the *gist*, whether it be a cityscape, a beach scene, or a domestic interior (Oliva and Torralba, 2006). But to fill in the details (and to possibly correct an initial misimpression) my gaze must shift from region to region in the scene, identifying agents and objects and clarifying their relationships or interactions. In architecture, the process of constructing a design is not constrained by a pre-existing scene, but the cognitive processes are similar: a first idea of the whole may guide the search for details; the attempt to mesh the details may necessitate changed notions for the pieces which may in turn propagate to affect the design of the whole. And this interaction of bottom-up and top-down design may proceed through many iterations.

> Construction is the art of making a meaningful whole out of many parts. ... I feel respect for the art of joining, the ability of craftsmen and engineers ... the knowledge of how to make things.

A crucial difference between visual perception and architectural design is that in a visual scene the "pieces" are already there (though what pieces and details we attend to, and what relations we emphasize is open to the varying goals of perception within the action-perception cycle), whereas in architecture the very building blocks may change as design proceeds – but always constrained by the architect's understanding of available materials and the skills needed to assemble them. Whether in architectural design or in making sense of our immediate environment, the interaction between the overall gist and the filling in of details must yield a representation that can guide our action appropriately. Probing these processes – from imagination and perception to construction – poses many challenges for neuroscience whose solution will enrich, and be enriched by, the conversation with architecture.

Meanwhile, Back in Singapore

Let me close with the work of another architect, Richard Hassell, who practices in Singapore. He is one-half of the architectural firm WOHA – the WO is Wong Mun Summm and the HA is Richard Hassell, and they founded this practice about 20 years ago. From http://www.world-architects.com/en/woha/ we learn that "WOHA combines awareness of local context and tradition with an ongoing exploration of contemporary architectural form-making and ideas." Some of their work has links to the eco-architecture of Ken Yeang as exemplified in their 2013 Singapore hotel PARKROYAL on Pickering, shown in Fig. 10, bringing the greenery into the design of the building, both for aesthetic and functional purposes.

When asked about WOHA's East-West connections, Hassell says "We follow a more 'Eastern' way of putting buildings together – complexes and compounds rather than objects, blurred lines between inside and outside, facades that relate to textiles and woven surfaces rather than solid forms." But in the rest of this section, I want to review the themes of Hassell's TEDx talk, "Making Density Great - a toolkit for 21st century cities," https://www.youtube.com/watch?v=swcgJYbuJ7s.

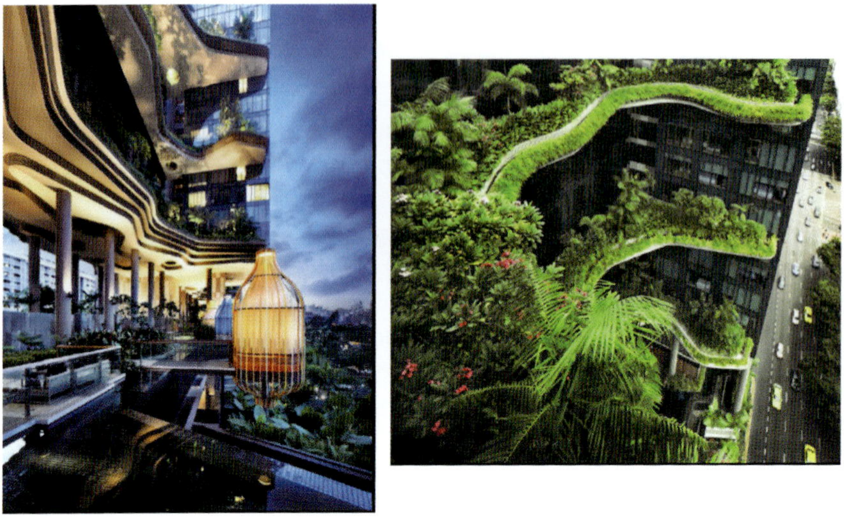

Fig. 10. WOHA's PARKROYAL on Pickering hotel in Singapore.

We are now at a transition point in many places in Asia and South America and Africa where we have new city structures springing up as people flood in from the countryside. What is the city of the future to be like if it is to be a more livable place than a collection of shantytowns? One answer is to house people in vast tracts of tall buildings where, at least, access can be provided to basic utilities like electricity and water. Yet in New York and Chicago, there have been disasters where such high-rises have become places in which people feel warehoused with no sense of community, and they become a breeding place for crime. Hassell's solution is again eco-architectural. We get a clue from the right side of Fig. 10 where we see greenery not as something to plant in the grounds of a building but as something which can be integrated into the building at multiple levels, so that even in a high-rise the tenant is connected to greenery nearby, bringing open space rather than isolation into their high rise living. Indeed, the floors between two successive levels of greenery can form a village in which people can build a community, with open walkways allowing neighbors to greet each other, a far cry from the ill-lit long corridors of the New York and Chicago developments.

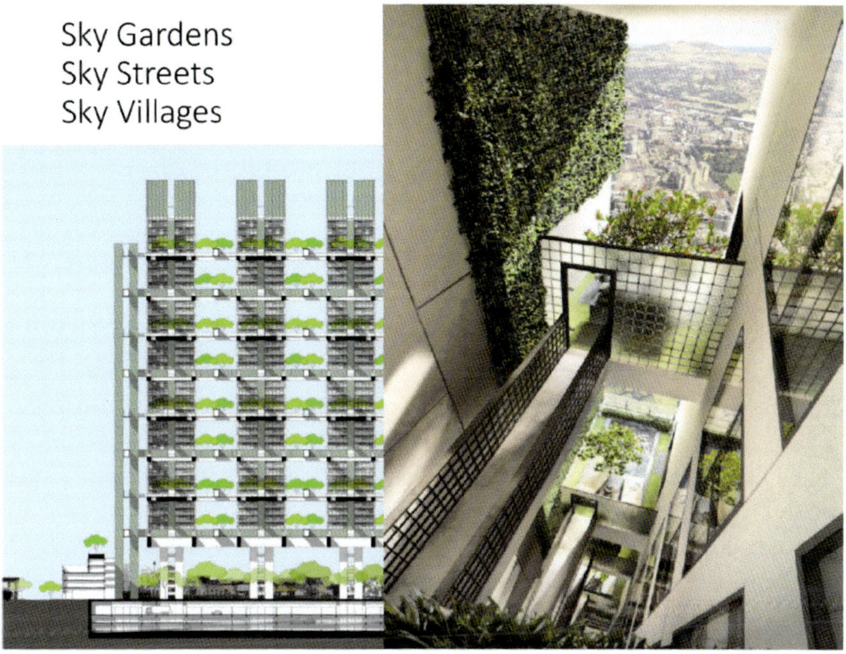

Fig. 11. Sky Gardens, Sky Streets, Sky Villages. (Courtesy of Richard Hassell)

On the left of Fig. 11 we see a schematic view of a skyscraper designed such that in every five floors, there is public space with greenery; at right is an image of the view looking down through the openings between levels. The result is that tenants in this huge skyscraper have a "sky village" that provides a community rather than an anonymous existence.

A Good Life, Revisited

And so we return to the question – "What defines a Good Life?" We may include creature comforts and well-being as an individual touchstone, and these can be enriched by the presence of beauty. Beyond this immediate impact on the individual there is the need for a sense of community and identity, of individual freedom wrapped up in individual challenge. What constitutes freedom and what defines community cannot be easily labeled as East versus West, though it is very much bound up with cultural patterns. Do you want to be free as a member of a particular democracy or as a member of a striving new society or as a member of a religious faith or ...?

We have seen how architecture can engage in the construction of a good life, and learned that in many cases architectural decisions are political decisions, and may be strongly influenced by the decision as to whose good life the built environment is to serve. Different buildings lead us to think about the good life in different ways and I've tried to show how the interaction between the culture and the cognition and brain processes of the individual occupant or the individual architect offers a promising start and exciting challenges for the development of a neuroscience for architecture.

An important point has for now been implicit: this traffic beyond boundaries must be of interest to both parties. Neuroscientists will engage with architects not only as a form of "translational science," where architecture rather than medicine provides the challenges for applications of neuroscience findings, but conversely the architects must pose questions that stimulate new basic research on cognition and the brain without demanding that every such effort has an immediate practical payoff.

References

Arbib, M. A. (1989) *The Metaphorical Brain 2: Neural Networks and Beyond*, New York: Wiley-Interscience.

Arbib, M. A. (2003) Rana computatrix to human language: towards a computational neuroethology of language evolution. *Philos Transact A Math Phys Eng Sci*, *361*(1811), 2345-2379.

Arbib, M. A. (2012) Brains, machines and buildings: towards a neuromorphic architecture. *Intelligent Buildings International*, *4*(3), 147-168. DOI:110.1080/17508975.17502012. 17702863.

Arbib, M. A. (2013a) Neurons, Schemas, Persons and Society—Revisited. In G. Auletta, I. Colagè and M. Jeannerod (Eds.), *Brains Top Down: Is Top-Down Causation Challenging Neuroscience?* pp. 57-87, Singapore: World Scientific.

Arbib, M. A. (2013b) (Why) Should Architects Care about Neuroscience? In P. Tidwell (Ed.), *Architecture and Neuroscience: a Tapio Wirkkala - Rut Bryk Design Reader*, pp. 42-75, Espoo, Finland: Tapio Wirkkala Rut Bryk Foundation.

Arbib, M. A. (2015) Towards a Neuroscience of the Design Process. In S. Robinson and J. Pallasmaa (Eds.), *Mind in Architecture: Neuroscience, Embodiment and the Future of Design*, pp. 75-98, Cambridge, MA: The MIT Press.

Arbib, M. A., Billard, A., Iacoboni, M. and Oztop, E. (2000) Synthetic brain imaging: grasping, mirror neurons and imitation. *Neural Networks*, *13*(8-9), 975-997.

Arbib, M. A. and Bonaiuto, J. J. (2012) Multiple Levels of Spatial Organization: World Graphs and Spatial Difference Learning. *Adaptive Behavior*, *20*(4), 287-303.

Bartel, T. (2013) Buddhas, Todai-Ji Temple, Nara, Japan. *Photo of the Day, Unesco World Heritage Sites*, https://travelpast50.com/buddhas-todai-ji-temple-nara-japan/.

Bennett, H. (2013) The Psyche of the Library: Physical Space and the Research Paradigm. Art Documentation: *Journal of the Art Libraries Society of North America*, *32*(2), 174-185.

Bennett, H. (2014) *Buildings with Brain Power: Library Architecture in Neural Terms.* Paper presented at the Session 149 - Art Libraries with Science and Technology Libraries - at IFLA WLIC 2014: Libraries, Citizens, Societies Lyon, France.

Bermudez, J., Krizaj, D., Lipschitz, D., Debborah, D. and Nakamura, Y. (2014) fMRI Study of Architecturally-Induced Contemplative States. *Abstracts of the 2014 Conference of the Academy of Neuroscience for Architecture, https://drive.google.com/file/d/0B2w6wLfWBCccUU5NWkJCZ1pmb1k/view?pref=2&pli=1,* 18-19; Video at https://www.youtube.com/watch?v=ipcuDil11jYA.

Bonaiuto, J. J. and Arbib, M. A. (2014) Modeling the BOLD correlates of competitive neural dynamics. *Neural Networks, 49*, 1-10.

Cahn, B. R. and Polich, J. (2006) Meditation States and Traits: EEG, ERP, and Neuroimaging Studies. *Psychological Bulletin, 132*(2), 180-211.

Campbell, J. W. P. and Pryce, W. (2013) *The Library: A World History*. Chicago: Chicago University Press.

Carlson, L. A., Hölscher, C., Shipley, T. F. and Dalton, R. C. (2010) Getting lost in buildings. *Current Directions in Psychological Science, 19*(5), 284-289.

Cliff, D. (2002) Neuroethology, computational. In M. A. Arbib (Ed.), *The Handbook of Brain Theory and Neural Networks, 2nd edition* (pp. 737-741). Cambridge, MA: The MIT Press.

Eberhard, J. P. (2008) *Brain Landscape: The Coexistence of Neuroscience and Architecture*. Oxford, New York: Oxford University Press.

Fagg, A. H. and Arbib, M. A. (1998) Modeling parietal-premotor interactions in primate control of grasping. *Neural Netw, 11*(7-8), 1277-1303.

Gibson, J. J. (1966) *The Senses Considered as Perceptual Systems*. Boston: Houghton Mifflin.

Gibson, J. J. (1979) *The ecological approach to visual perception*. Boston: Houghton Mifflin.

Guazzelli, A., Corbacho, F. J., Bota, M. and Arbib, M. A. (1998) Affordances, Motivation, and the World Graph Theory. *Adaptive Behavior, 6*, 435-471.

Hart, S. (2011) *EcoArchitecture: the work of Ken Yeang*. Chichester, UK: Wiley.

Jeannerod, M., Arbib, M. A., Rizzolatti, G. and Sakata, H. (1995) Grasping objects: the cortical mechanisms of visuomotor transformation. *Trends Neurosci, 18*(7), 314-320.

Kornberg, K. (2014) *Research without Borders*: Jonathan James and Waldemar Kaczmarski.

Lelin, Z., Chi, Y. M., Edelstein, E., Schulze, J., Gramann, K., Velasquez, A., . . . and Macagno, E. (2010) Wireless physiological monitoring and ocular tracking: 3D calibration in a fully-immersive virtual health care environment. *Engineering in Medicine and Biology Society (EMBC), 2010 Annual International Conference of the IEEE*, 4464-4467.

Lieblich, I. and Arbib, M. A. (1982) Multiple Representations of Space Underlying Behavior. *The Behavioral and Brain Sciences, 5*, 627-659.

Maguire, E. A., Nannery, R. and Spiers, H. J. (2006) Navigation around London by a taxi driver with bilateral hippocampal lesions. *Brain, 129*(11), 2894-2907. doi: 10.1093/brain/awl286.

Maguire, E. A., Woollett, K. and Spiers, H. J. (2006) London taxi drivers and bus drivers: A structural MRI and neuropsychological analysis. *Hippocampus, 16*(12), 1091-1101. doi: 10.1002/hipo.20233.

Neisser, U. (1976) *Cognition and Reality: Principles and Implications of Cognitive Psychology*. San Francisco: W. H. Freeman.

Neutra, R. R. (2014) On the Past and Future Tensions Between Documentation and Esthetics in Architectural Photography *Arts, 3*, 335-349; doi:310.3390/arts3030335.

O'Keefe, J. (1983) Spatial memory within and without the hippocampal system. In W. Seifert (Ed.), *Neurobiology of the Hippocampus* (pp. 375-403). New York: Academic Press.

O'Keefe, J. (2014) Spatial Cells in the Hippocampal Formation. *Nobel Lecture on 7 December 2014 at Aula Medica, Karolinska Institutet in Stockholm*, http://www.nobelprize.org/mediaplayer/index.php?id=2413.

O'Keefe, J. and Dostrovsky, J. O. (1971) The hippocampus as a spatial map: preliminary evidence from unit activity in the freely moving rat. *Brain Research*, *34*, 171-175.

Oliva, A. and Torralba, A. (2006) Building the gist of a scene: The role of global image features in recognition. *Progress in brain research*, *155*, 23-36.

Pallasmaa, J. (2009) *The thinking hand.* Chichester, UK: John Wiley & Sons.

Pallasmaa, J. (2012) *The Eyes of the Skin: Architecture and the Senses 3rd Edition*: Wiley.

Robinson, S. and Pallasmaa, J. (Eds.). (2015) *Mind in Architecture: Neuroscience, Embodiment, and the Future of Design*. Cambridge, MA: The MIT Press.

Scoville, W. B. and Milner, B. (1957) Loss of Recent Memory After Bilateral Hippocampal Lesions (Reprinted in J Neuropsychiatry Clin Neurosci 2000, 12, pp. 103-113). *J. Neurol. Neurosurg. Psychiatr.*, *20*, 11-21.

Squire, L. R. and Wixted, J. T. (2011) The Cognitive Neuroscience of Human Memory Since H.M. *Annual Review of Neuroscience*, *34*(1), 259-288. doi: doi:10.1146/annurev-neuro-061010-113720.

Szentágothai, J. and Réthelyi, M. (1973) Cyto-and Neuropil Architecture of the Spinal Cord. In J. E. Desmedt (Ed.), *New directions in electromyography and clinical neurolophysiology*, *Volume 3* (Vol. 20-37). Basel: Karger.

Turvey, M. T. (1992) Affordances and prospective control: an outline of the ontology. *Ecological Psychology*, *4*, 173-187.

Turvey, M. T. and Shaw, R. E. (1978) The primacy of perceiving: An ecological reformulation of perception as a point of departure for understanding memory. In L.-G. Nilsson (Ed.), *Perspectives on memory research: Essays in honor of Uppsala University's 500th anniversary*, pp. 167-222, Hillsdale, NJ:: Lawrence Erlbaum Associates, Inc.

Ulrich, R. (1984) View through a window may influence recovery. *Science*, *224*(4647), 224-225.

Zeisel, J. (2006) *Inquiry by Design: Environment/Behavior/Neuroscience in Architecture, Interiors, Landscape, and Planning (Revised Edition)*. New York: W. W. Norton.

Zumthor, P. (2012) A way of looking at things. In P. Zumthor (Ed.), *Thinking Architecture, Third, expanded edition*. Basel: Birkhauser.

8 The Good Life Lost and Found: East, West, Home's Best

Svend Erik Larsen

School of Communication and Culture,
Department of Comparative Literature,
Aarhus University, Denmark

Yangtze River Chaired Visiting Professor,
College of Literature and Journalism,
Sichuan University, China
litsel@cc.au.dk

Conditions for a Good Life

One of the many Syrian refugees who are now crossing Europe has ended up in Denmark, at least for the time being, without knowing if he can stay or has to move on. Asked by a journalist from a Danish news channel about his life in Syria he said: "You only know what a good life is when you have lost it." - "Did you have a good life back in Syria? - "Yes," he said. "Anyway, it was a comfortable life. But perhaps a good life is simpler than a comfortable life. Now I have to reinvent it somehow, somewhere. I don't know if it is possible. I'm here alone without my family."

Perhaps a quote from John Michael Coetzee's novel *Diary of a Bad Year* (2007) can clarify the basic simplicity he is looking for. In the novel a disillusioned old writer is composing small reflections for a German anthology, including one on J.S. Bach's music. He imagines how he would have addressed the old master:

> "In the name of all mankind, please accept these words of tribute, inadequate though they are, and let all you endured of those bitter last years of yours, including the cruel surgical operations on your eyes, be forgotten." [...] In naming him, do I name the father I would elect if, from all the living and the dead, one were allowed to elect one's father? Do I in this sense choose him as my spiritual father? And what is it that I want to make up for by bringing at last a first, faint smile to

> his lips? For having been, in my time, such a bad son? (Coetzee, 2007: 221-222).

Apparently, this is not about a good life, at least not about the life of a desperate refugee. And yet. The old writer regrets the misery of Bach's late life and his own role as a bad son – a loss of a good life for both. He also envisions what a good life should contain. First, it should embrace a sense of three interconnected levels of identity: (1) identity as a human being – he writes on behalf of all mankind; (2) social identity, in this case as a member of a family, real or symbolic, (3) personal or individual identity – the possibility to select and define one's own identity and family affiliation. Second, a good life should offer the possibility to be reinvented by being recontextualized once it is lost, even on the limit of the impossible. He experiences Bach's music as an example of such a transformation: the personal misery is transposed to music that elevates others with joy and excitement. At the same time he also mobilizes his own capacity to imagine new vistas in life close to the impossible – what if I forget the past and imagine I can invent a new human, social and personal identity by electing a new father? Impossible, of course, but not when understood as a way of imagining a new origin or a new beginning. What is lost may be reinvented by a radical use of the imagination. Third, for the three entangled levels of identities and the transformations to work they have to activate a synthesis of intense emotional and rational engagement, here presented as the joyful absorption in the music together with a reflexive imagination of a new life.

Well, the writer is sitting comfortably at his desk in Adelaide, Australia, saddened by a misguided life which is now nearing the end. The refugee is confronted with a more radical destruction of the possibilities for a good life. Coming from a warzone of unspeakable horrors he is, of course, searching for safe survival which had earlier been a self-evident part of his comfortable life. Yet, he realizes that this is not enough for a good life. We may say that safe survival is a *necessary* condition for a good life, while the three other aspects, shared by the writer and the refugee, indicate the *sufficient* conditions for a good life: (1) the three interconnected levels of identity, (2) the belief that it is possible to recreate a new beginning leading to a good life, (3) the integration of emotional and rational capacities in that endeavor.

I will claim that the necessary and sufficient conditions are universal and transcultural conditions for a good life. However, a good life always unfolds in particular cultural and historical contexts where it is charged with a cultural and historical specificity. Across cultures, the concrete contextualization produces a cultural differentiation with regard to the meanings and practices of identity, of reinvention and change of a good life, of the synthesis of emotion and rational thinking involved in the process, and of survival in safety. Such meanings and practices constitute what I will then call culturally specific cognitive patterns of the sense of a good life, in this paper just 'cultural patterns' for short, and I see them primarily as cultural patterns of identity formation. I use the term 'cognitive' in a broad sense to mean 'concerning the mind', and when I combine 'meanings and practices' I want to stress that cultural patterns generate practices and are changed by the practices they shape and thereby make the meanings of a good life a dynamic and contextual part of culture.

In some cases, such patterns may show extensive overlaps, typically within larger regions like Asia or Europe; in other cases, they may expose so many differences that they become almost contradictory and trigger cultural animosities as we see today when global flows of migrants and refugees often clash with local and indigenous cultures. More than ever, we are aware that identities defined by religion, often expressed in terms of collective values of honor and shame, do not easily marry with identities shaped on secular grounds emphasizing individual rights, initiative and responsibility. The capacity to change one's own life and the surrounding society may be evaluated in positive terms and encouraged in an individualized Western culture, but not so in a honor-based structure such as, for example, the Indian caste system or other hereditary social formations; the separation of emotional from intellectual patterns in a scientific world view may be hard to unite with cultures where meditation or religious faith is appreciated as a fundamental way to connect to the world at large.

The Syrian refugee tries to escape a conflict between a good Western-style comfortable life as an urban professional and a brutal dictatorship as well as the conflict between Sunnis and Shias. Moreover, he is about to meet yet another sense of good life in what is for him a remote corner of Europe – a welfare state with a reduced importance of the family, a family which is also different from the tradition of an extended family which is a broadly accepted basis of the good life where he comes from. He has been subject to war crimes and crimes against humanity that dissolve the whole cultural pattern of a good life in the rubbles of Aleppo. His sense of human, social and personal identities and their interconnection is radically disrupted, any clear possibility of transformation to another life has vanished and the paramount fear and despair block any rational planning of a way out, except for an escape to some place where the conditions for a good life perhaps can be met.

Probably, he would better understand Cynthia Ngewu than Coetzee's writer. She is one of the victims of apartheid where her son was brutally killed, now being urged to forgive her tormentors during the deliberations of the South African *Truth and Reconciliation Commission*. She has experienced the same radical break down of cultural patterns for a good life as the Syrian refugee. Being invited to express herself face to face with her son's killer, her life is safer than during apartheid, but also far away from what the Syrian remembers as a comfortable life. Yet, she is now trying to reinvent the possibility of a good life on the new local post-apartheid conditions by using a coping strategy, reconciliation, which is not available to the refugee during his present tribulations and of no interest to Coetzee's protagonist.

> "This thing called reconciliation ... if I am understanding it correctly ... if it means this perpetrator, this man who has killed Christopher Piet, if it means he becomes human again, this man, so that I, so that all of us, get our humanity back ... then agree, then I support it all." (Krog, 1999: 164).

Beyond the individual and contextual difference between the writer, the refugee and the apartheid victim, the quotation shows that the same conditions for a good life are at stake. First, the three intertwined dimensions of identity: herself, the others and humanity; then the synthesis of an emotional investment, revealed in the broken syntax of her declaration, and an intellectual grasp of the situation she tries to understand 'correctly'. Finally, and most importantly, she is trying to reconnect to the conditions for a good life by way of a transformative coping strategy, reconciliation which, perhaps, will allow her to transcend her sufferings.

When war crimes and crimes against humanity have caused havoc, the cultural pattern supporting a good life loses its power and specificity. Yet, at the same time attempts to renew the conditions for a good life make the basic features of cultural patterns for a good life, their potential overlaps and their differences more visible. That is why the experience of radical wrongdoing will frame this paper. The ambiguous experience of homecoming will set the context, and reconciliation confronted with gross violations will define the focus, while the East-West relation will be redefined, opening a final perspective.

Homecoming

Since Homer's *Odyssey*, coming home after the war has been cherished by the assumption that the warriors or refugees came back to the good life they had known. However, already the *Odyssey* casts doubt on precisely that idea: Ithaca was close to a collapse. This doubt has not been reduced throughout the centuries. Only rarely did the good life look as the returnees imagined it and perhaps it was not even there in the first place. All of it was an idealizing illusion that had evolved during the hardship away from home. The notion of nostalgia captures this problem (Boym, 2008). The term comes from renaissance medicine as a name for a psychosomatic aberration in soldiers, a painful relation to the lost good life back home (cf. Hutcheon, 1998). Today, this condition is known by countless veterans under the label PTSD, while the term nostalgia itself has evolved into a general term for a sentimental longing for the good old days when the conditions for a good life were supposed to be self-fulfilling.

Today the dubious blessings of homecoming have further been questioned by the fact that many diasporic communities simply have no home to return to in terms of a nation or a homeland: the Kurds, the Palestinians, the Cossacks. Others have only recently acquired a home, but as a contested place: Jews in Israel or peoples in postcolonial nations. Other home grounds have been fragmented after a short existence: Yugoslavia, The Soviet Union, or, alternatively, united after a short division: Germany or Vietnam, all of which generates doubt about what home actually is. And some people, like the Syrian refugee, have left destruction behind that probably will last throughout their lifetime whether they leave or stay as Cynthia Ngewu does. So, home may offer an ideal image of the good life, but in real life it is mostly a fragile construction that shatters the conditions for a good life and exposes a host of cultural differences in ways of coping with its vulnerability. Nowhere is a good life a state of affairs, but an ongoing process that requires coping strategies to overcome the broken equation that is supposed, automatically, to identify home with a good life.

This situation will become apparent in a few photos, all depicting the return of hostages from war zones atrocities. Against all international rules of war they could have been killed or executed by their captivators. One would expect that the reaction across the world to the freeing and the return of the surviving hostages would be one of happiness and jubilation. But it is not so, although the extreme situation is the same for all: war crime and crime against humanity. Yet, without denying that the situation is extreme, both the radical transgression and the homecoming are evaluated differently in different cultural contexts: for the captivators the atrocities are a legitimate response to the wrongdoing inflicted upon them by their enemies; for the hostages and their home culture the opposite holds. My three cases balance on the limits of different cultural patterns, and this positon exposes more clearly the complexity of cultural encounters and the mutual challenges they face when the good life is defined and realized.

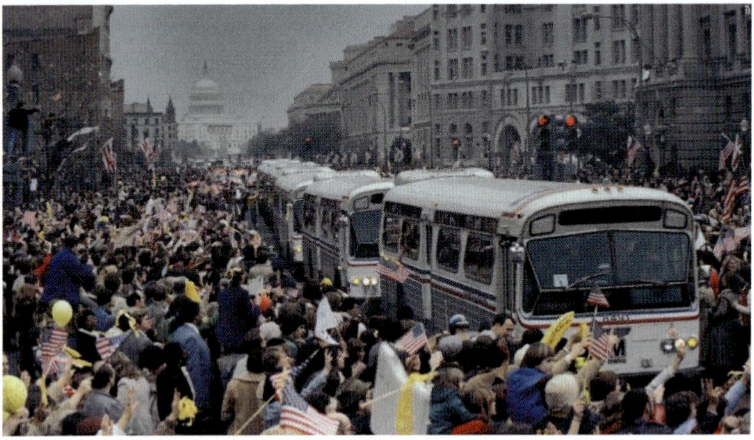

Fig. 1. American hostages returning from Iran in 1979.

The first photo shows the return of the 52 hostages from the American embassy in Iran, after 444 days during 1979 to 1981 and after the failed rescue expedition under the Carter administration. They were received as national heroes, boosting the national solidarity in the USA. No one was really interested if a ransom or any other symbolic price had been paid for their release, and the humiliation of the USA caused by the abortive rescue was silenced. Instead reports of the hardship endured by the hostages created an emotional sense of solidarity with the hostages who had sacrificed themselves for their country and lived up to highest standards of American identity. Back in Teheran the anti-American feelings were strengthened and the students holding the captives and the hardliners were applauded. There was pride and jubilation on both sides, and the rift between East and West was intensified: each party indulged in their own national agenda, and both sides vilified their opponent and saw the other as having committed unforgivable acts. The two incompatible official stories are, one, that the Americans returned to the good life they had left, and, two, that the Iranians demonstrated their power to define a good life for themselves, liberated from Westernized influence.

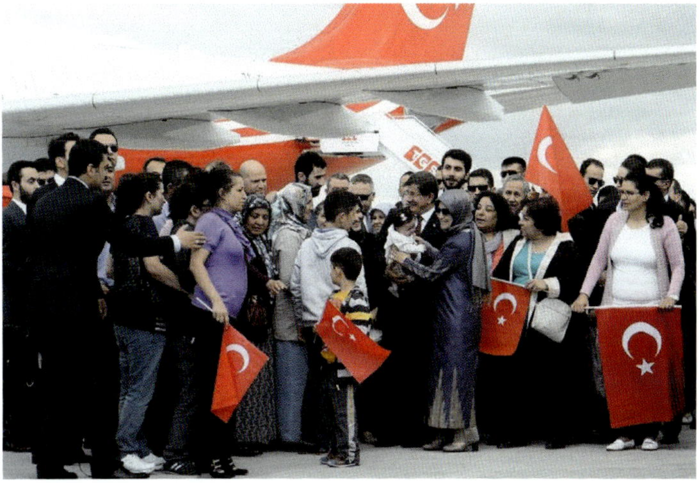

Fig. 2. Turkish hostages returning from Islamic State in Iraq 2014.

The second photo is from September 2014 when two groups of Turkish hostages, a group of diplomats in Northern Iraq and a group of truck drivers, were set free after having been captivated by the Islamic State. Here the conflict unfolds within the Muslim world between a more or less secularized Turkey, still belonging to Islam but ambiguously turned to the West, and Islamic fundamentalists of the Sunni persuasion claiming to recreate the caliphate with a good life based on the sharia. The Turkish government, on the photo represented by Prime Minister Ahmet Davutoglu at the center, vehemently denies having negotiated a price for the approximately 80 people. An admission would have forced it to acknowledge that it had not adhered to its own principles of never caving in to terrorists. As in the first case, both sides regard the actions of the other as unforgivable and the sense of justice in the general public was satisfied by the emotional engagement in the release of the two groups, ignoring the political aspects of dubious negotiations or any wider political context, including the internal conflict between Sunnis and Shias and between fundamentalism and secularization that are also present in Turkey itself. Also these hostages returned home to a good life in Turkey, opposed to the life under sharia. The same structure as in the American case is repeated, but with a different content. Now, the state took the price and the pride, not the individual heroes.

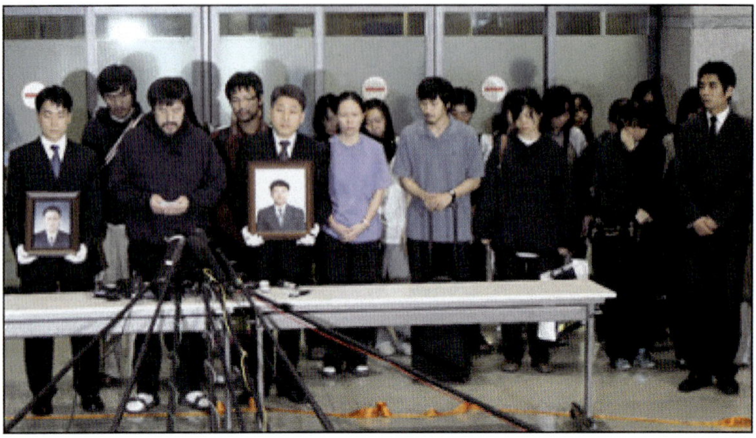

Fig. 3. Korean hostages returning from Taliban in Afghanistan 2007.

The third photo also depicts a recent event, from 2007, but it is a much more complex case without the clear dichotomous structure of the previous ones. A group of about 20 Korean hostages returned from captivity under the Taliban where two of them had been killed. No jubilation was displayed, at least not in public. Instead, a somber group bowed and cried in front of the Korean people, the government and their own families as an expression of their contrition. They had brought shame on them all by going to Afghanistan and letting themselves be humiliated by being captured, a humiliation which then was transferred to the whole nation. For all, the event had produced a profound shame and sorrow including, to make matters worse, the national government which had been forced to humiliate itself to work for their release through negotiation. Yet, the government adamantly denied any concession to the terrorists, thereby saving face and honor on behalf of all Koreans. The families tried to recompense the loss of honor by making excuses to the nation on behalf of the returning family members. In a Korean perspective, the most unforgivable acts are committed by the hostages, not the Taliban.

The 21 persons were Christian NGOs on a charity mission they had planned and carried out themselves. As Christians they naively believed that the universal principle of helping others and the emotional motivation for such acts were universally acknowledged values. Instead, they were accused of trying to convert Muslims. Conversion is a mortal sin, *shirk*, for Muslims. The Korean reaction at home was different from the international reactions from fellow Christians which were based on universal principles that were neither endorsed by the Koreans nor the Taliban: the Pope appealed to the Taliban on the basis of Christian mercy, Christian communities prayed around the world, and some governments made appeals to the perpetrators with reference to universal human rights and to various international principles. Thus, the homecoming makes East meet West in several precarious ways: Christianity vs Islam; traditional Korean honor code vs an international reference to universal principles for human interaction; individual responsibility for choosing to do what is right vs collective responsibility for nation and family.

The Westernized cultural pattern based on universal human rights did not exercise any influence on the sense of justice in Korea or Afghanistan. The hostages are guilty, not innocent, and the role of the Taliban is not important for the Koreans. What the rebels did to the NGOs is precisely what could be expected when people against all reason seek them out to the detriment of the honor of the nation and the family. Hence, the dishonorable details of high level negotiations must be denied, publicly and vehemently, in order to protect the collective code of honor. The act of the hostages was transgressive and unforgivable according to the local cultural pattern for a good life, and the negative effect of their expedition was amplified when the return added public visibility to their behavior. The only applicable coping strategy was public confession of guilt, not, as in Cynthia Ngewu's case, an attempt at reconciliation, overcoming the guilt of the perpetrators. The returnees were not regarded as heroes like the American or as innocent victims like the Turks, but as culprits. The acts of the Taliban – like those of the Islamic State – are also unforgivable, and transgressive, but only according to universal human rights principles of Western origin, not to their own standards and not important to the Koreans. In contrast to the two previous cases, we see the limits of the tools with which a local cultural pattern for a good life can cope with transgressive acts in a modern globalized context. In all three cases, different as they are, negotiating cultural patterns is out of the question. East and West, home is not always the best.

Cultural Patterns of Identity

Before I return to the complexity of the Korean case and show how it emerges in Yi Mun-Yol's novel *An Appointment with My Brother* (1994), I will present a few concepts and methodological principles for the study of cultural patterns from the point of view of their limits and for the understanding of the difference between East and West. The study of cultural patterns across cultures invites two different approaches. One of them focuses on the center of such patterns in an attempt to describe their constitutive core features from within. This approach rests, often implicitly, on the assumption that specific cultural patterns can be understood intrinsically as immanent and closed structures. The capacity to change is not part of their make-up. On the contrary, changes are often regarded as the influence of external threats and, hence, evaluated negatively. Contradictorily, culture is studied in a way that makes its historicity a secondary feature.

In this perspective East meets West means to be exposed to either the 'yellow danger' or Western depravation, and as Rudyard Kipling famously announced: 'never the twain shall meet'. The corollary is that in principle different cultures may live side by side without any mutual exchange, either because they actually do not interfere with each other or because the most powerful define the relevant cultural patterns of the cultural communities they dominate. In this perspective, and as we know from the European and non-European colonial history across the world, the subordinate cultures are regarded as inferior. In other words, when describing each culture in its own immanent specificity, it is tacitly assumed that this is the way they actually unfold.

However, this type of cultural studies does not correspond to the actual conditions and life of any culture, least of all in the contemporary globalized world. Here, it is evident that cultures do not just co-exist in the same space, but that they blend and mingle. Hence, it does not suffice to know about other cultures from the outside, but to imagine what it means to live another culture which is not only placed in front of my doorstep but inhabits my own house where migrants may live in the room next to mine. Actually, cultural patterns have always negotiated and changed in a mutual and not always friendly exchange with none of them being sure to keep the upper hand, not even the colonizing culture. But this negotiation has never been seen as constitutive of the intrinsic nature of a culture, but just as a secondary activity, often undertaken reluctantly. However, in a globalized world the growing need for a multicultural process of exchange has been intensified by multiple and intersecting migratory flows – from tourism, business, education and research to waves of refugees from war, suppression or poverty.

This situation requires another approach to the study of the various cultural and cognitive patterns engaged in cultural encounters. My suggestion is that we no longer should look at cultures primarily from their intrinsic built-up, but from their liminal zones where they not just happen to overlap, but where they must overlap. It happens when they are faced with a shared experience none of them can cope with alone but nevertheless have to cope with, particularly in cases when the limits of a culture and its sustainability are radically and violently transgressed as in the stories of the hostages.

To explore cultures from their limits and their capacity to cope with transgressions and thus redefine themselves amounts to understanding cultural patterns with the aim of opening them to a mutual exchange with other patterns. This approach does not define fixed core values as the central aspect of cultures, but precisely its potential openness that emphasizes dynamic cultural exchanges as the core function of cultures, and makes visible the challenges and the potentials as well as the difficulty and necessity of encounters. In this perspective, the good life does not rest on the immanent cultural pattern of identity, but on the capacity to master an ongoing negotiation with alternative patterns. In the American and the Turkish examples, this capacity is completely suppressed in the public space; in the Korean case the uneasy feelings triggered by the homecoming call for it but in vain.

To pursue such a study we need to introduce a filter between the basic and transcultutural conditions for a good life and the particular cultural pattern that shape the meanings and practices of a good life in local cultures. This filter is the culturally specific distinctions between right and wrong. Otherwise the meaning of a *good* life cannot be negotiated. The distinctions unfold on three levels:

(1) the legal (right or wrong according to a legal system)
(2) the ethical (right or wrong according to ethical norms)
(3) the anthropological (right or wrong according to a conception of what is human or non-human).

These levels are underpinned by two basic dimensions:

(1) A *metaphysical* dimension that legitimizes the basic distinctions between right and wrong which allow each of the three levels to function as overarching principles within the culture. This dimension may have a religious foundation as in the majority of local cultures around the world, or it may be based on secularized universal ideas of humankind as in the case of human rights that attempt to define basic translocal conditions for a good life. Such principles can be made explicit in religious

dogmas, constitutions, codes of law, mythologies or in various contracts, treaties and declarations, all with a kind of formal status. They explain what is right and wrong in a local culture but also what is regarded as the most radically transgressive wrongdoing – offending the gods, God, the Prophet or the ancestral spirits or, alternatively, committing crimes against humanity. This type of trespass may be labelled unforgivable, and in the context of the patterns discussed in this paper it means any act that is considered as a radical destruction of the conditions for a good life (cf. Derrida, 2001, Neiman, 2002).

(2) A *cultural or social* dimension which is a non-formalized sense of justice. In general terms the sense of justice is the ethical-emotional agreement shared by a larger or smaller cultural community that transforms informal and invisible norms into deliberate human action charged with human responsibility. The sense of justice is historically contextualized and interacts with and underpins the formal legal system in the culture where it operates (cf. Walker, 2007: ch 1). On the grounds of local traditions, then, the sense of justice is the shared acceptance or rejection of distinctions between right and wrong and their social consequences, like the fairness of a verdict, the validity of social duties, gender relations or the shared sense of what humans may or may not do to each other. However, a sense of justice does not work according to explicit principles but according to shared and locally accumulated everyday practices that unite what is seen as possible rational actions and acceptable emotional reactions to events.

If the distinctions between right and wrong are challenged, the basic principles that support them may turn out to be incompatible with the sense of justice that translates them into social practice. This will be the moment that marks the radical transgression of the cultural pattern. A case in point is the seriousness of rape cases in India that caught global attention in December 2012 when a girl died after being gang-raped in a bus in New Delhi. The formal law, based on English colonial rules and European individual civil rights and universal human rights, was clear. But there is a long tradition in India for turning the blind eye to rapes in order not to disrupt a local sense of justice, mainly based on the caste system although it is formally abandoned. The death penalty was also a legal option, but could not be issued because of India's ratification of human rights, whereas it is accepted by the local sense of justice, but again derived from the caste system, not from the universal legal principles of European based law (see http://en.wikipedia.org/wiki/2012_Delhi_gang_rape_case).

Whether a verdict would be regarded as fair or not was defined, on the one hand, by the caste system were the whole matter depended on who are the perpetrators and who are being raped, and the code of honor and shame which is built into this traditional social hierarchy. For some, the woman got what she deserved, and also indirectly brought it upon herself, by her dishonorable behavior of travelling in the evening only accompanied by a fellow student with whom she had no family relations. On the other hand, women groups and all who were opposed to the effects of the officially disregarded caste system and referred to universal human rights principles were in support of strong punishments, even a death sentence.

We may easily say that rape is unforgivable, but what is unforgivable or not is debatable in the local cultural context where an age-old tradition-based sense of justice competes with a formal law, inherited from colonial times, implying a more recent sense of justice based on individual human rights including women's rights. Some of the positions originate in the East, others in the West, and some of them blend indiscriminately East and West. This is a context that makes necessary an approach for the study of cultural patterns in a transcultural perspective focusing on their limits where competing patterns meet.

Coping Between the Universal and the Local

Reinventing the conditions for a good life after having been subject to radical wrongdoing requires coping strategies that allow the victims and their societies to leave the broken tools behind and shape new ones to reestablish a cultural pattern for a good life (Minow, 1998, Walker, 2007, Larsen, 2012a, 2012b). The quote from Cynthia Ngewu's testimony to the *Truth and Reconciliation Commission* about reconciliation is such an attempt where reconciliation or forgiveness is staged collectively as a coping strategy of the post-apartheid society in order to enable people to overcome the consequences of radical transgression.

Considering their disastrous enormity it is often assumed that gross violations evoke an immediate universal agreement on the horrific nature of the events, not least because they are now disseminated by the global media and embodied by the millions of refugees many of us meet face to face where we live. Moreover, it is also assumed that a universal sense of how to cope with them could be found to help people rebuild a good life after the all-pervasive breakdown of the cultural norms they live by. Since the aftermath of WW2, reconciliation entered as an important component of transitional law (see http://ictj.org) and also in international courts and transnational models for reconciliation commissions. The South African commission suggested a particular notion of forgiveness as such a coping strategy and tried it out in practice with a global resonance. (cf. Bois and Bois-Pedain, 2008).

However, more often than not the contrary happens, in South Africa as well (cf. Wilson, 2001). In situations of gross iniquities we clearly see that the same experience or events perceived from different cultural perspectives are also evaluated differently. In some cases extreme violations are perceived as going beyond the legally, ethically and anthropologically determined values of any given culture in ways that challenge their religious or overall secular foundation and defy the local sense of justice, ultimately destroying the conditions for a good life.

However, at the same time and in a competing cultural perspective, such events are also proclaimed to be right in all their horrific aspects as in the present day Islamic State and earlier in the South African apartheid regime and during Pol Pot's rule in Cambodia. Also, the use of torture is defended by some as necessary and thus legitimate to prevent a superior evil-like terrorism, as it happened during the Bush administration although it goes against both American law and the sense of justice of the majority of Americans. In short, the type of transgression and the strategies of coming to terms with them are so different that they more than anything else expose *both* the limits and shortcomings of otherwise self-evident and traditional cultural patterns *and* the relativity of the universalized attempts to restore cultural sustainability. Thus, universal human rights are not accepted or ratified worldwide nor are the international courts they have fostered, not even among Western countries where universal human rights originated. Liminal situations like these display the vulnerability of cultural patterns around the world and the need for them to negotiate with other patterns to cope with radical wrongdoing. Here, suggestions of universal coping strategies such as forgiveness constitute only one option. Even if such strategies succeed in replacing other and more local metaphysical underpinnings of legal, ethical and anthropological building blocks of a good life, they cannot replace the non-formal sense of justice that is a basic condition of cultural cohesiveness bound as it is to age-old traditions.

This asymmetry between the universal and the local is made particularly clear when gross iniquities emerge in cultures and societies in transition – like South Africa after apartheid, the European countries after the dismantling of their empires, Europe and Asia after WW I and WW II, China after the cultural revolution and the reforms, Korea after the Korean war that has never formally come to an end. Here, there is no agreement, not even within the countries, of what are radical transgressions and how to cope with them, nor is there agreement when an external or foreign influence is added to break the deadlock, which today will always be added – due to media, trade, travel, migration, international politics, etc. Some events are too earth shattering to be coped with by the formalized value systems of a culture in a way that both satisfies the metaphysical underpinning of right and wrong and the sense of justice framing the sustainability of everyday life as a good life. Iniquities on that scale defy any formalized reaction: to give the South African torturer Eugene de Kock 212 years in prison for his atrocities probably makes good formal sense and satisfies basic legal principles, but it does not produce a sense of justice, because no practical meaning can be attached to it. New practices are required to enable people to imagine future collective and individual identity formations.

In this context, coping strategies offer different solutions: healing practices in cultures with shamans, sacrifices to the gods, revenge, praying, alternative medicine, revolution, prayer, legal prosecution, confessions, ritual practices, ritualized punishments. But basically, coping is of two kinds: *retribution* or *reconciliation*. Retribution or retaliation is about redressing the balance after serious wrongdoing by paying back in terms that are accepted as equivalent to the crime – an eye for an eye (Miller, 2006). In contrast, reconciliation is about recontextualization through negotiation in order to unlock a fixed situation and reinstall a balance on new conditions. In retributive practices the reaction to a devious act is defined entirely by the context of the violation that caused the retribution and, hence, the reaction is absorbed by the past. In contrast, practices of reconciliation are instead defined by the agents or subjects involved in reconciliation, not by the event, and are directed to their future actions (Griswold, 2007). The agents have to mobilize their imaginative power to recontextualize the event in a future-oriented perspective (cf. Tutu, 1999). Any sense of justice is based on those two principles.

The coping strategies I am preoccupied with belong partly or entirely to reconciliation. Coping as reconciliation may be defined as a deliberate cultural reaction to radical wrongdoing that draws on the power and the media of imagination directed toward the future. By doing so, coping recontextualizes radical wrongdoing within a context to be determined by those involved in the act of forgiveness and offers the possibility of a shared reworking of emotions and memories related to the event.

One such reconciliatory coping strategy which has gained a universal status is forgiveness, not least through a series of truth and reconciliation commissions on different continents that built on universal human rights principles. Investing forgiveness in a negotiation between cultural patterns of identity requires, first, that it is de-universalized and seen as a historical and culturally specific coping strategy with its own limitations. Forgiveness is not a universal model based on de-contextualized universal features, but a component that must be modified in a local context as it has itself been remodified since its ambiguous emergence in early Christianity. Without being aware of its historical specificity the application of forgiveness will lose a necessary contextual sensitivity and it will be turned into yet another example of cultural hegemony, colonial or otherwise. There are two ways of indicating the limitations of forgiveness as a coping strategy – one has to do with the historicity of the concept itself within Western culture, the other with the cultural complexity of the situations beyond that context where it may be used.

The Historical Context

The basic writings and notions of Christianity emerged in a double context: on the one hand, a linguistic context defined by Greek culture that seeped into the early biblical texts simply because they were written in Greek (although the spoken languages to a large extent would have been Aramaic and Hebrew); on the other hand, equally important was the institutional, cultural and political Judaic culture under Roman colonization where the Law and the rituals it prescribed were central. No wonder that the early attempts to formulate a Christian notion of forgiveness show some ambiguity. The two essential features are the following:

(1) *Unconditionality*: forgiveness does not require contrition as in Islam or Judaism where forgiveness also plays an important role, but based on confession and remorse. In Christianity, confessing one's sins is a noble gesture, but not a prerequisite for forgiveness. "Father, forgive them, they do not know what they

are doing" are the words of Christ in Luke 23:34. It is an act of mercy bestowed upon humankind by God and also preached as a model for humans in their relations with each other while judging, and hence forgiving the more serious trespasses committed against God lies only in his hands. However, certain sins are unforgivable, even at the end of times, repentance or no repentance (Matthew 12:31-32, Mark 3, 28-29, Luke 12:10). Hence, unconditionality is neither unambiguous nor unlimited.

(2) *Universality*: Universality means that forgiveness embraces all humans, both believers and non-believers, although Saint Paul who first launched the idea of universality, only zooms in on Jews and non-Jews. In more general terms, forgiveness disregards social and ethnic hierarchies, a wide ranging idea that becomes central to Christian preaching. Yet, already to begin with, to write religion out of established institutions and social hierarchies and make it a message to everyone was an audacious new idea. Focusing first on the distinction between Jews and non-Jews shows that this idea always will have to confront the specific institutions and hierarchies in any given cultural context. Universality cannot avoid being contested by the limitations of forgiveness as a specific cultural practice.

Ambiguous or not, the insistence on universal and non-hierarchical unconditionality undid the notion of the unforgivable as defined by Judaism, namely disobedience of the Law and its endless series of regulations of daily life. In that sense forgiveness redirects the sense of justice defined by the Jewish community from the Law to the reality of everyday life.

However, in order to have a wider dissemination this new understanding was formulated in Greek, a language that did not possess an adequate notion or terminology to formulate the new ideas (Keene, 1995, Konstan, 2010) The standard Greek term for a similar type of coping with wrongdoing, namely pardoning, is *syngnome* (Romilly, 1979). This is the type of mercy that may be unconditional, but is not universal and it is hierarchical. It is the merciful gesture of the sovereign towards his subjects, often bestowed arbitrarily which is not in the power of the subject to perform. Like gift-giving in many cultures, it is a self-assuming demonstration of power dressed up as tolerance and generosity. The term *syngnome* is not used in Saint Paul or in the gospels, but this understanding of pardon still lived on Christian culture

(Perrin, 1987). In Saint Paul, who was active around 60 CE, the terms used to make the new type of forgiveness understandable is a metaphor of economical origin, *charizomai*, meaning to give freely without counting on any return or profit.

In the Gospels, composed around 50 years later, the favorite term for forgiveness is most often *aphesis* (the verb is *aphiemi*). It means 'release', 'remit from debt or from legal bindings', 'send away'. This is the word Jesus takes up repeatedly in his teaching and parables and also uses in the Lord's Prayer. Two different but similar Greek terms (used in the tragedies) are *luo* and *eleuthero*. However, they are not used in the Gospels, although their meaning approaches that of the verbal forms of *aphesis*. However, *apo-luo* (the prefix *apo-* makes it stronger and more concrete) is used on a few occasions (cf. English 'apology'). It means 'send away, 'set free' and, in particular, 'divorce' (cf. Matthew 19: 3-10) or 'release from captivity' as in the case of Barabbas in front of Pilate. When Barabbas, probably a murderer, is chosen to go free instead of Jesus, the verb used is *apoluo*.

Yet, it is most often the economical register that is used in the Gospels to specify what it means to be forgiven – to be set free from any debt. Surprisingly, forgiveness as the primary reconciliatory practice is presented without having its own terms, but is defined as a negation of the economical sense of balance which follows the logic of retribution. When forgiven, one is supposed *not* to pay back. It is therefore a concept that constantly invites to have its context redefined to provide the negative term with a positive sense. The sense of justice that forgiveness is supposed to establish against Greek and Roman paganism as well as against Jewish dogmatism is deeply influenced by the local complexity of conflicting cultural patterns of its time, no different from today's blended globalized cultural environment of religious beliefs and ethical values. Forgiveness is born as a notion about negotiating and transcending competing and incompatible cultural patterns.

However, during the following centuries a de-contextualized and universalized notion of forgiveness emerged to make it a powerful non-ambiguous component of Christian dogmatism. This attempt was reinforced by the institutionalization of the Christian church where confession became a sacrament with a well-defined practice exacting out, retributively as it were, the payment for particular everyday sins in number of prayers and candles. With the expansion from Palestine and Rome to the rest of Europe and later through missionaries and colonial expansion to the rest of the world the universal status of forgiveness was reasserted by its global outreach, influencing the judiciary, ethics and anthropology wherever it went, often in blatant conflict with local conceptions of the unforgivable and of the local sense of justice.

However, this situation changed, first with Protestantism and then more strongly with European Enlightenment in the 18th century. Gradually, the universal religious content acquired a different but equally universal underpinning, namely the secular idea of a universal human nature that generated universal human rights, which later influenced the judiciary, ethics and anthropology across the globe by pushing its Christian origin into the background. Now, the foundation of forgiveness as a universal coping strategy is human emotions, namely a universal human capacity to empathize with all other human beings beyond cultural differences. Forgiveness, modelled after the Christian notion, is seen as a universal human capacity that eventually, this is the vision, will create a world society of world citizens in peace and harmony (cf. Hunt, 2007, Larsen, 2014). The practice of forgiveness, supposedly based on a naturally given potential for empathy, is then a universally valid ethical obligation for all humans toward any fellow human being, not the prerogative of a merciful God.

In this way, forgiveness became part of a huge civilizing project on European grounds. Essential for the sense of justice, it gave rise to the conception that each human being is held accountable for individually intended and actualized actions based on the assumption that the emotional constitution of people is a transcultural human constant. Therefore, this sense of justice came to be seen as potentially unifying global notion – no reference to fate, to class, to caste, to community, to original sin, to rebirth, to collective norms derived from honor or shame, to local histories, etc. As long as this universalizing endeavor works on the level of formal law, political organization or in the curricula of colonial education, it proved to be successful, also outside Europe. However, the moment forgiveness as a moral principle and a coping strategy against mischievous acts had to work on the level of a local sense of justice, the confrontation with the diverse, context-bound, historically developed, religiously grounded senses of justice was unavoidable. It never worked between slaves and slave owners, between colonizer and colonized, between antagonistic tribes and families or between classes. As in the Indian rape case, forgiveness then revealed its own contextually determined limitations.

If a reactivation of forgiveness has a potential today in a globalized world where local cultures are globalized as well, it will have to be accepted as a particular coping strategy with no claim to universality. It will have to engage with local reconciliatory coping strategies and to counterbalance retributive components of local senses of justice. Then forgiveness may promote a negotiation between different cultural patterns. To reflect its limitations and its possibilities, unconditionality and universality will have to be supplemented with three more features that points to its contextualization:

(1) *Remembrance*: Forgiveness is a way of remembering, not of forgetting as the popular misunderstanding will have it. Forgiveness only works when the wrongdoing is recalled loud and clear. This happens through a recontextualization, for example from the torture chambers of apartheid to the hearing venues of the *Truth and Reconciliation Commission*, or, as in the confession in the Catholic Church, from the norms of everyday life to the measurement spelled out by the church. The negotiation that forgiveness opens is a negotiation concerning an agreement about the new context where coping can take place. Forgiveness could be called remembering through recontextualization.

(2) *Speech act*: Forgiveness has to be a speech act, mutually recognized by the parties involved, or to be established through non-verbal signs that can be translated into verbal language. To forgive silently or silently tell oneself that I am forgiven has no meaning. As a speech act forgiveness is similar to a verdict or a confirmation of a contract, hence the rich use of legal and economical metaphors in the context of forgiveness in both Saint Paul and the Gospels. Being bound to language also means that forgiveness depends on local semantics and the problems of translation.

(3) *Continuity*: In contrast to a verdict, forgiveness is not a one-off; it is performed as a continuous or repeatable process. Forgiving today and hating tomorrow has no meaning. That is why forgiveness has to be integrated as a coping strategy in tune with the inbuilt inertia of a local sense of justice, which unfolds as a daily process or is used as a compass for everyday normative behavioral habits over time. Forgiveness is not a conclusion, but a possible beginning to a process which, as process, may give rise to a good life – again.

With such additions, forgiveness offers a coping strategy in cases of serious iniquities that have destroyed the conditions for a good life and broken down the cultural pattern that guides its meanings and practice. Here, its proclaimed unconditionality and universality are filtered through its historical specificity and limitations. What these features actually emphasize is that forgiveness offers a broader perspective than that of the local context where it is applied – unconditional means it is not conditioned by this context alone and universal means it is applied with a view to other cultural patterns outside the troubled context. In this way forgiveness may be turned into a concrete practice of negotiating between cultural patterns by insisting on recontextualization beyond the shattered context, on verbal dialogue and on conditions for a continuous dialogical process. In contrast to the Christian promise of God's forgiveness, this context-sensitive redefinition does not guarantee redemption. It all depends on the people involved. When Desmond Tutu was invited to visit Israel and Palestine to see if something similar to his *Truth and Reconciliation Commission* would be possible, he returned to South Africa: "They are not ready yet".

Homecoming: Mission Impossible?

Yi Mun-Yol's novel *An Appointment with My Brother* (1994) questions this readiness. The story is about the first meeting of two brothers in a small Korean enclave in China, Yenji, neither North nor South and not a unified Korea either, still separated as it is by the unfinished war between North and South. The wider context is the cultural pattern of the old united Korea and Asian ideas of ethics and personal identity based on family, honor and shame. It is shared by the brothers, but is also contradicted by communism and capitalism which now mark the opposition between North and South which, in turn, is challenged by the overlapping of Christianity, paganism and Buddhism in both Koreas. Here, as in the case of the Korean hostages, a code of honor and shame is a core component of the cultural pattern (cf. Peristiany, 1965). Whether the home of the brothers is the North or the South, the cultural pattern they rely on to cope with the disasters that have hit the nation, the family and the individual lives is imbued with contradictions.

The tenor of this mixed choir of normative voices, surrounding the hostages as well as the two protagonists of the novel, is self-control. Public show-off of emotions, courage, or failure is not appreciated. This attitude is a mental make-up generated by Buddhism and Confucianism dating back much longer than the actual division of Korea. In fact, silence and secrecy is more important than public exposure, not just as a pragmatic necessity when dealing with matters of national security, but as a question of honor and shame. Publicity may lead to a damaging loss of face to which a spectacular retaliation would just add shame to be shared by individuals and families alike and maybe the community at large. The homecoming of the hostages showed that provoking the loss of face of the government and the families is a more radical wrongdoing than the actual killing of some hostages. In order to divert the attention from those losing face, the returning hostages take the blame on their own shoulders. Silence is best, indirectness acceptable, directness shameful, no matter the cause (Alford, 1999). This is a shared feeling across Asian cultures that share the ethics of Buddhism and Confucianism. In *Men of Evil* (2013), James Dawes explains the fate of the returning Japanese war criminals after WW II:

> When Kaneko-san returned to Japan after release from China, he was publicly shamed – not for the war crimes he committed, but for confessing to them.[…] Nobody wanted these things to be said. Men like Kaneko-san and Sakakura-san were violating the collective decision to be silent and to deny. And for that too they could not find forgiveness. (Dawes, 2013: 195-196)

This confusing blending of Korean traditions with the contemporary Asian context, with Christianity, secularism, a post-colonial situation and globalized warfare together with the conflict between capitalism and communism defines the complex cultural space of *An Appointment with My Brother* and the conflicting cultural patterns the two brothers have to deal with in order to come to terms with the past, cope with the unforgivable acts they remember, and turn to the future.

The two half-brothers embody the division of the country: the narrator Yi Hyeonseop, about fifty years old, from Seoul, and Yi Hyeok, in his forties, from the North. Their encounter takes place over a couple of days in a Korean borderline region in China, a political, national, geographical, legal, cultural as well as a spatial limbo. What unites them now is their recently deceased father to whose spirit they both want to pay respect by traditional offerings of food and drink from his home in the South. In the 1950s the father defected from the South as a militant communist, leaving his wife and two children behind in poverty, remarried in the North and fathered three younger children. Both feel partly cheated by their father. The Southerners felt that their loss was caused by the family in the North who took the father away physically; in contrast, the Northerners blamed the Southern family, feeling that the eldest son left behind nevertheless was always first in their father's mind. The father being the head of both families according to the tradition embodies the double blame for the loss of a good life on both sides. Because of his constitutive role in the family, the father has acted in an unforgivable way. Now he has died from cancer.

At first, the two Yi brothers are hesitant to talk about their own social lives. If they did, they may either appear shamefully unsuccessful or force one brother to lose face because of the other's achievements. So they discuss general family matters instead. In accordance with old traditions, the family name, Yi, is maintained in both families, and we learn that it is a prestigious name from the old united Korea. Being the eldest son, the brother from the South is responsible for the rituals to be carried out and, as is appropriate, he also took the initiative to organize the encounter and paid for his Northern brother's illegal visit to Yenji. Instead of deciding whether the funeral should be Christian, Buddhist, Confucian or agnostic they agree to perform the customary ancestral rites together in the neutral limbo of Yenji, but facing North Korea. This is a matter of honor for both.

To begin with, both brothers are full of stories of pride from their respective homes and past lives. If they revealed any real troubles, they would inevitably lose face and honor and thereby also betray their homeland and family or, alternatively, they may embarrass the brother as a member of the larger family. They are in a deadlock, both feeling that radical wrongdoing was committed by their father to both halves of the family, and that the family is the only thing that keeps them together through their name and the shared ancestral worship. It is not the war or devastating later results of ideologically motivated conflicts that are first in their minds as radical wrongdoing. It is what happened within the family as a breach of its honor code when the father defected. Gradually, it transpires that the father was not a hero in the North, but was excluded from society as a suspicious renegade from the South, and also that the brother from the South turned out to have earned a great deal of money in dodgy speculations and ends in the novel by smuggling antiques back home via a dealer that lurks around him in the hotel in Yenji.

At a certain point the masks begin to fall, helped by heavy drinking that transports them beyond any sense of shame or of losing of face in front of each other. In Yenji, they are not in the ancestral home of the father which they should have returned to for the paternal service. And luckily so. The home in the South would have belonged more to the senior than to the junior brother. But in the limbo where they actually meet neither of them is more at home than the other. This is made clear during the ritual they perform – facing the North with a sacrifice of food and drink from the father's birthplace in the South. This situation of forced spatial mediation, as it were, allows the brothers, step by step, to reveal the complexity of their real lives in the two parts of Korea, and their prejudices about the other Korean region begin to dissolve. Their mutual compassion and empathy becomes stronger than the deep-rooted honor and shame and the public prejudices on each side of the armistice line.

However, when they eventually sober up, they cannot verbalize this development. Such a concession would mean a loss of face. It has to be indirect. So, the quasi-forgiveness that unfolds between them is communicated to the reader by a narrative strategy of double articulation in which the I-narrator, Hyeonseop, verbalizes his emotional recognition of the brother's predicament and wishes to reach out to him in empathy. In contrast to the ancestral rite, an open act of forgiveness would still be too norm-breaking and they are almost incapable of finding a verbal expression. I render the decisive steps in italics:

> "Please give my love to my brothers and sisters." Then I added, *like one who has made a grave decision*. "And *our mother*, too."
>
> One of my anxious uncertainties after I decided to meet my brother was how to call my brother's mother. Should I call her "mother in the North?" Or "my stepmother?" But none of them seemed appropriate. So, I had been making do with "your mother." But she became "our mother" in my mind at the moment of parting from my brother.
>
> In ancient Oriental law, there were exceptional cases where a second legal wife was authorized by law. To my modern *rational sensibility*, too, my brother's mother was fully entitled to be regarded as my mother. But I was surprised that "our mother" *rolled out of my mouth* so naturally, and started. My brother was *visibly affected*, too. His alcohol-clouded face sobering up at once, he gazed at me for a moment and bowed.
>
> "Please, give my love to my sister and my nephews and nieces. And to *our mother*, too."
>
> "Our mother" seemed to *roll out of his mouth* quite naturally, too. (Yi, 2002:81-82).

As the context requires, the process of forgiveness is highly complex. It happens through an exchange of gifts, mutual bows and words of greetings before they depart. The process is rendered in a mixture of an interior monologue of questioning and of explicit dialogue; moreover, the narrator's voice activates the ancient cultural pattern of Korea beyond the personal and national divisions, called 'ancient Oriental law'. Before they met, both brothers have projected the effect of the wrongdoing of their father on their own half of the family and made it a victim. By paying respect to the dead father, they now both transcend that feeling, and the indirectly expressed mutual forgiveness is addressed toward the other brother and his family on which the sense of wrongdoing was projected. This is an attempt to recontextualize the wrongdoing from the past family, embodied by the dead father, to the present split family, embodied by the two living brothers. Forgiveness is a reconciliatory move from the dead to the living. It embraces the two families and regards them as one in the future; it also transcends the division of their two countries by reactivating a sense of justice below the radar of the official ideologies. In this move the two mothers become one mother by the use of an identical phrase, 'our mother', and by the narrator's identical way of describing the speech act: 'roll out of the mouth.' Taking into account the traditional Korean equivalence between mother, or woman, and nation (Hübinette, 2005), the exceptional nature of the brothers' exchange is clear. It is furthermore supported by the inserted information from the narrator on the role of a Korean wife. Beyond the family, they have a united Korea in mind.

In the new context of their present encounter only the indirectness of speech and supplementary facial expressions are available to the brothers. However, the narrator, coming from the South, also notes his own 'modern rational sensibility' which is built on explicitness. With this reference he shows an emerging awareness that explicitness may constitute the next step in the ongoing process of forgiveness, made possible by the recontextualization from the dead to the living. Due to the necessary indirectness at this stage of their relationship, forgiveness is not a finalized act, but it may initiate an emotional learning process once they have returned. In a sense, they have come home to the good life as a sense of family in accordance with the traditional cultural pattern that shapes the meanings and practices of a good life – in Korea at least. But they still live in separate worlds. As for the hostages, for them it is also a pattern with no fixed abode.

East-West Perspectives

Taken at face value, East and West indicate two localities. North and South do the same and other oppositions on the gyroscope as well. Division lines such as these may have some relevance in geopolitical terms, although they are still too simplistic. However, when we talk about cultural patterns shaping a good life they are less than helpful to produce an understanding of identity formations and a good life in a globalized world of dynamic cultural encounters. A sharp separation of East from West does not hold in the way Kipling envisioned in the heyday of European colonialism. And even back then it may have been the colonizers' wishful thinking; the empire had already started to strike and write back. Wars in Afghanistan are not new.

Rather than a place, the West is better identified with a translocalism, based first on a European and later on an American expansionism that transformed local cultural patterns in the image of the Western life style and a good life, ready to be universalized on a global scale. The receptiveness to this pattern all over the world, in the growing urban areas in particular, is evident. The one-child policy of mainland China in particular has helped create a huge urban class of young individualized consumers for whom the good life has its origin in a Western cultural pattern far removed from traditional Confucianism and collectivity of a communist leaning, and for the most part this sense of a good life is identified with what the Syrian refugee in Denmark pointed to as his comfortable life back in Syria. Hence, it is not located in the West but in Beijing, Shanghai, Aleppo and elsewhere. People living their daily life there have no difficulties going abroad and then coming home. The difference is manageable and not always noticeable. Until recently, the agenda for the cultural encounter between East and West has predominantly been defined by the Western cultural pattern, where the local cultural patterns rooted in a longer history appear as modifications of the Western pattern.

Whether the balance is tipping or not, Western expansionism has stopped, the global acceptance of its universalized cultural patterns is contested from East, West, North and South and it has been relocated again to the West and evaluated as a particular sense of a good life, mainly the life of an urban middle class. What is important now is, first of all, to be able to combine, blend and negotiate the potential of different cultural patterns. Today, many cultural patterns with a clear local origin and no immanent expansionist drive are nevertheless disseminated across the world to new locations through media circulation, trade and flows of people. In this context, East and West are poles in just one opposition among several others around the globe, each of them a blend of many influences, none of them pure and none of them understandable as intrinsically defined patterns for meanings and practices. This is a message the returning hostages should have brought with them to USA, Turkey and Korea and also the message they should have been told when they returned. But this did not happen.

Contrary to the attempts to support the negotiation between cultural patterns runs a strong tendency to retreat to the old self-indulgence in a world of sharp dichotomies between autonomous cultural patterns. The hostages exemplify this trend without noticing it or without the tools to transcend it, the Syrian refugee and the gang-raped Indian woman are victims of it, while Cynthia Ngewu tries to transcend it through reconciliation. Today, the following two global cultural patterns shaping a good life are competing and not eager to reconcile themselves: the good life is seen as a life that gives us the tools to negotiate changing encounters between different cultural patterns; or, the good life is seen as a life within the enclosure of a local cultural pattern. This opposition is far more important than the opposition between East and West and also more dangerous than the East-West dichotomy has ever been. Just ask the Syrian refugee.

References

Alford, C. F. (1999) *Think no Evil. Korean Values in the Age of Globalization.* Ithaca: Cornell University Press.

Bois, F. du and Antje, du B.-P., eds. (2008) *Justice and Reconciliation in Post-Apartheid South Africa.* Cambridge: Cambridge University Press.

Boym, S. (2008/2001) *The Future of Nostalgia.* New York: Basic Books.

Coetzee, J. M. (2007) *A Diary of a Bad Year.* London: Vintage.

Dawes, J. (2013) *Evil Men.* Cambridge: Harvard University Press.

Derrida, J. (2001) To Forgive: The Unforgivable and the Imprescriptible. *Questioning God*, John Caputo, Mark Dooley and Michael Scanlon, eds. pp. 21-51, Bloomington: Indiana University Press.

Griswold, C. L. (2007) *Forgiveness. A Philosophical Exploration.* Cambridge: Cambridge University Press.

Hübinette, T. (2005) The Nation is a Woman: The Korean Nation Embodied as an Overseas Adopted Korean Woman in Chang Kil-su's *Susanne Brink's Arirang. Intersections: Gender, History and Culture in the Asian Context* 11, August 2005. (http://intersections.anu.edu.au/issue11/hubinette.html) (Feb 29 2016).

Hunt, L. (2007) *Inventing Human Rights.* New York: Norton.

Hutcheon, L. (1998) Irony, Nostalgia, and the Postmodern (http://www.library.utoronto.ca/utel/criticism/hutchinp.html) (February 23, 2016).

Keene, F. W. (1995) Structures of Forgiveness in the New Testament (http://www.faithtrustinstitute.org/resources/articles/Structures-of-Forgiveness.pdf) (March 16 2013).
Konstan, D. (2010) *Before Forgiveness. The Origins of a Moral Idea.* Cambridge: Cambridge University Press.
Krog, A. (1999) *Country of My Skull.* London: Vintage.
Larsen, S. E. (2012a) After the Battle. Complexities of Emotional Post-War Reactions. *Repräsentation des Krieges,* Søren Fauth, Kasper Green Krejberg and Jan Süsselbeck, eds. pp. 355-369, Göttingen: Wallstein.
Larsen, S. E. (2012b) Forgiveness as a Challenge to the Law. *Dialogues on Justice,* Helle Porsdam and Thomas Elholm, eds. pp. 141-159, Berlin: de Gruyter.
Larsen, S. E. (2014) Emotion and Forgiveness in Literature. *Exploring Text and Emotions,* Patrizia Lombardo, Lars Sætre and Julien Zanetta, eds. Aarhus: Aarhus University Press. 63-89.
Miller, I. W. (2006) *An Eye for an Eye.* Cambridge: Cambridge University Press.
Minow, M. (1998) *Between Vengeance and Forgiveness. Facing History after Genocide and Mass Violence.* Boston: Beacon Press.
Neiman, S. (2002) *Evil in Modern Thought.* Princeton: Princeton University Press.
Peristiany, J.G., ed. (1965) *Honor and Shame. The Values of Mediterranean Society.* London: Weidenfeld and Nicolson.
Perrin, M., ed. (1987) *Le pardon.* Paris: Beauchesne.
Romilly, J. de (1979) *La Douceur dans la pensée grecque.* Paris: Belles Lettres.
The Bible (2001) *The Holy Bible* (ESV). Wheaton: Crossway.
Tutu, D. (1999) *No Future Without Forgiveness.* London: Rider.
Walker, M. U. (2007) *Moral Repair. Reconstructing Moral Relations after Wrongdoing.* Cambridge: Cambridge University Press.
Wilson, R. (2001) *The Politics of Truth and Reconciliation in South Africa. Legitimizing the Post-Apartheid State.* Cambridge: Cambridge University Press.
Yi, M.-Y. (1994/2002) *An Appointment with My Brother.* Seoul: Jimoondang Publ. Comp.

Links:

Delhi gang rape: http://en.wikipedia.org/wiki/2012_Delhi_gang_rape_case (Feb 29 2016).
International Center for Transitional Justice: http://ictj.org/ (Feb 29 2016).

Photos:

1) Return of US hostages from Iran, 1979 (http://edition.cnn.com/2014/10/27/world/ac-six-things-you-didnt-know-about-the-iran-hostage-crisis) (Feb 24, 2016).
2) Return of Turkish hostages from ISIS/Iraq (http://www.nytimes.com/2014/09/21/world/middleeast/dozens-of-turkish-hostages-held-by-islamic-state-are-freed.html) (Feb 23, 2016).
3) Return of Korean hostages from Taleban/Afghanistan (http://www.thegatewaypundit.com/2007/09/afghan-report-taliban-raped-korean-hostages-over-over/) (Feb 23, 2016).

9 A Good Death: Resolving the Complexity of Mortality

Andy Hau Yan Ho[*] and Geraldine Tan-Ho[†]

*Division of Psychology,
School of Humanities and Social Sciences,
Nanyang Technological University, Singapore
andyhyho@ntu.edu.sg
†LifeLAB Institute; HCA Hospice Care, Singapore
geraldinetan@lifelab.sg

Introduction

Among all complexities of the world, there lies one that is ever so clear yet opaque, so obvious yet convoluted, that it brings confusion, disillusionment and even fear to the brightest of minds. Throughout our existence, human beings have long attempted to resolve the complexity of mortality. From the practices of Alchemy to the search for the Fountain of Youth, kings and empires across the East and the West have devoted their lives to finding the one potion that can give them eternal life, to save them from the dread of old age, and to survive the finality of death.

Despite millenniums of efforts, not a single soul has succeeded in this seemingly fruitless endeavor. Yet, the quest for immortality continues until this day and age, as top scientists across the globe are actively and vigorously trying to conjure a new Elixir of Life. Through harnessing the exponential power of computing and information technologies, inventor and futurist Ray Kurzeil has predicted that by the year 2045, the human race will reach the tipping point of *Singularity, "an era in which our intelligence becomes non-biological and trillion times more powerful than it is today"* (Kurzeil, 2005), enabling us to transcend our physical limitations, allowing us the impossible prospect to live infinitely in the rim of intelligent machines.

While the jury for Singularity, the most newfangled offering of eternal life, awaits the test of time, the majority of us still die biologically, psychologically, emotionally and spiritually as we reach life's end. At least to this very day, death remains the only certainty in a life time filled with uncertainty; an inconvenient but undeniable truth. But despite the fact that every human being will experience death *(a known constant until proven otherwise)*, either through dying or vicariously through the loss of a loved one, death remains a shadowy figure that most people have difficulty facing, discussing or even considering. In between our fear and avoidance towards mortality and our unceasing and futile pursuit of immortality *(again, a known constant until proven otherwise)*, we have relegated death to the periphery of our lives, to keep it out of sight and out of mind. And in doing so, we inevitably become victims of our own fear as we turn weak and powerless in the face of dying, death and bereavement.

Having experienced countless mortalities over the past decade through our work in end-of-life care settings; having witnessed first-hand the dread and desolation of the dying and the bereaved due to a death denying culture; having encountered the grief and sorrows of hospice and palliative professionals under an oppressive healthcare system, and having advocated tirelessly for the promotion of holistic and dignified palliative care; it has become clear to us that we, as a people, desperately need to enhance our knowledge, understanding and emotional capacities in managing our own deaths, as well as those of our loved ones. It is based upon these observations, as well as our conviction to empower individuals to find meaning and solace in the face of mortality, that we begin this chapter. Our thesis will first examine the premise of a death denying ethos that has troubled our minds for the longest of time, followed by an exploration of the evolving attitudes of mortality in recent eras, and finally, a discussion on the imperative of public health palliative care for the promotion of *A Good Death*.

Premise of a Death Denying Ethos

If we are to offer a discourse that directs people towards a good life, we must also engage in a conversation that guides people towards a good death, life and death being intertwined. But such conversations have not been easy in the past, or in the present, as human beings have been entranced in a death-denying ethos, one that spans across the East and the West.

Philosophers and researchers have unceasingly argued that we as a species must balance between accepting and denying death in order to maintain a grasp on reality while remaining committed to a future limited by mortality. Death acceptance however has never been a forte of our species, as attitudes towards death and dying in modern societies have generally accentuated the scent of fear, anxiety and rejection. In his highly influential book *The Denial of Death*, anthropologist Ernest Becker established that, *"The idea of death, the fear of if, hunts the human animal like nothing else; it is a mainspring of human activity – activity designed largely to avoid the fatality of death, to overcome it by denying in some way that it is the final destiny for man"* (Becker, 1973).

Renowned sociologist Talcott Parsons had also observed that it is human tendency in *"bringing to bear every possible resource to prolong active and healthful life"* (Parsons, 1963), and only accepting the defeat of death when it is felt inevitable. He argued that the repugnant association between mortality and grief, *"not only in the sense of pain, but also in the frustration of disability and the various aspects of mental suffering"*, would cause people with fatal illness to mitigate and even numb their agony through widespread use of medical sedatives. The spiritual distress and existential anguish related to the end-of-life would inevitably lead individuals to emotionally distance themselves from the reality of death, creating a widespread phenomenon of apathy. Parsons (1963) further warned that the *"renunciation of the moral responsibility"* on mortality would ultimately conduce to the institutionalized provision of coping for the dying and the bereaved, as well as the *"complete dependence on higher authority"* in the occurrence of death.

Despondently, both Becker and Parsons forecasted a death-denying culture that negates and undermines the strengths of individuals, families and communities in facing, overcoming and governing the challenges of morality. Together they have forested a not too distant future where the experience of death and bereavement are oppressed and stigmatized.

Evolving Attitudes toward Death and Dying

In his seminal work, *Limits to Medicine: Medical Nemesis*, philosopher Ivan Illich asserted that human attitudes toward death and dying are determined largely by the prevalent social contexts, specifically its political economies, institutional structures, social actors and enduring myths (Illich, 1976). He further argued that the vision of a 'natural death' in old age with years of preceding good health is only a contemporary ideal, as the dominant image of death of every society is vitally linked to its prevalent concept of health.

While death has traditionally been deemed a *Spiritual Event* in ancient history, often linked to the divine act of God or of a higher power, and served as a pathway to eternal bless or eternal suffering in both Western and Eastern religious ideologies such as Catholicism and Taoism (Ho and Chan, 2011), Illich had observed a radical transformation of how society perceived mortality at the dawn of the 18th Century. The Industrial Revolution of the time had created unseen wealth as well as unprecedented social segregation between the rich and the poor. This critical paradigm shift marked by significant advancements in medicine allowed the wealthy to purchase health and to keep death away; yet, the deprived were often left for dead with the stroke of illness in an era that lacked institutional justice or established social welfare. During this period, medical care for protracting illnesses was deemed a mark of distinction, and the health of a nation became an obvious apparatus to ensure the economic productivity of its people (Foucault, 1973). However, without a social collective to instill policies that safeguarded population wellbeing, good health of children became a responsibility borne by parents; old age became a privilege defined through class and economic power; and death became an *Untimely Event* for those who were neither frail nor old.

By the 19th Century, doctors began to certify death as the outcome of specific ailment, their supremacy over health inevitably thrust them into the prestigious and powerful middle class. The prevalent belief and hope that doctors had the ability to control disease progression also gave rise to the myth that they had control over death, and hence the new elite status of the clinician. The expansion of medicine's jurisdiction also saw the proliferation of hospitals as well as the emergence of a new consciousness of the scientifically trained health professional. Under their gaze, the human body became objectified, whereby individuals were no longer perceived as social entities but as constellations of objects that were constantly under medical scrutiny. When death ceased to be spiritual but transmuted into medically identifiable germs and viruses, a *Timely Death* with clinical symptoms had become the ideal end-of-life scenario among the masses. This period marked the emergence of a health-denying culture, one that *"destroys the potential of people to deal with their human weakness, vulnerability and uniqueness in personal and autonomous ways… is the ultimate backlash of hygienic progress and consists in the paralysis of healthy responses to suffering, impairment and death"* (Illich, 1976).

Following extraordinary social development after the First and Second World Wars, the United Nations and the Universal Declaration of Human Rights were established, with the 20th century being celebrated by the germination of trade and workers' unions that uplifted the welfare of the working class. During this period, good health as well as good death through public health regimes and institutionalized medical care had become a service that society owed to all its members. This new image of mortality endorsed new forms of social control, where the state was now responsible for the proper deaths of all men and women, while deaths without appropriate medical treatment were liable to legal inquiries. As doctors and hospitals held increasing power and accountability for the health of ordinary citizens, individuals' responsibility and duty for upholding their own well-being diminished. The growing dependency on the medical profession had also created the *Clinical Death*, a spiritual vacuum in how people perceived and understood mortality. In the epoch of medicine dominance, death was converted into a scientific event controlled by doctors, so much so that deathbeds had moved away from homes and communities into hospitals and institutions, and the second offices of priests and pastors were taken over by nurses and clinicians. The medicalization of death had extended beyond the dying person to survivors, as grief has been identified as a form of psychological disease with specific symptomatology and management strategies (Engel, 1961). As such, the commodification of health had severely undermined *"the unique spiritual and intellectual strength of the human race which enables them to rise to the challenges of dying and death"* (O'Corman, 1998).

At the turn of the twenty-first century, medical knowledge and technology had reached unprecedented heights, stretching the human lifespan by an average of 36.7 years (Ham, 1994). Such increase in life expectancy was not without its cost, as the common stage of a *Mechanical Death* in modernity entails patients in critical conditions waiting helplessly and often unconsciously with heavy anesthesia for their final demise in the intensive care unit of hospitals. Often in today's advanced societies, individuals are no longer able to set the scene for their own deaths as the mandate of doctors and healthcare systems protect them from dying. The vast emerging body of research on death and grief had further transformed the personal and communal experiences of mortality into a public discourse where doctors and psychiatrists claimed authority. Yet, medical professionals often cannot agree among themselves about the finality of death as they continue to administer aggressive yet futile treatments to prolong life without realizing their power is nothing more than temporal (Sweeting and Gilhooley, 1992). In her landmark research that examined the psychosocial aspect of oncology care, Elisabeth Kubler-Ross revealed that hospital staff often withdrew from the bedsides of dying cancer patients because they did not have the capacity to cope with the emotional pain of death, let alone support patients in their final and most vulnerable moments (Kubler-Ross, 1970). Others have also observed that due to our obsession with living, we have gone to extraordinary efforts to conceal death, to use euphemisms such as 'passed away' or 'gone to a better place' to keep death at bay (Barley, 1995). Such fear and avoidance have subjugated meaningful dialogue on, acceptance of, or preparation for one's imminent mortality.

From a divine act of God evolving into an untimely event, a timely death, a clinical death and ultimately a mechanical death, the attitudes and perceptions towards mortality have transformed dramatically with emergence of the medical market. With increasingly accelerated progress in health technologies and pharmaceutical agents that focus predominately on curation, voluntary enslavements of personal health to the hands of doctors and the bureaucracies of healthcare institutions are now commonplace, leaving little or no room for human responsibility in the governance of death and dying (Conway, 2012). Evidently and regrettably, Becker's and Parsons' prediction of a death-denying ethos that oppresses the experience of mortality and loss have clearly been realized in the modern era.

The Rise of Public Health Palliative Care

Despite the apparent grim and oppressive outlook towards life's end, there is light, as well as hope, before the end of the tunnel. Led by Dame Cicely Saunders, a passionate group of healthcare professionals, who were committed to expand the narrow and limiting scope of curative medicine to include palliation and comfort support, initiated the modern hospice movement in the 1960s. Fueled by the ideals of 'total pain' and 'whole person care' (Sanders, 1967), these pioneers, together with succeeding generations of compassionate clinicians, nurses and social workers, have created and pushed forth a new regime of care for the end-of-life; one that does not aspire to prolong life nor hasten death, but focuses on palliative interventions for reducing the physical pain and controlling the bodily symptoms associated with dying, while emphasizing the alleviation of psycho-social-spiritual distress and suffering experienced by terminally-ill patients and their families via greater provision of holistic and compassionate support.

In 2004, the World Health Organization cemented the vital significance of palliative care and defined it as "*an approach for improving the quality of life of individuals and their families facing problems associated with life-threatening illness, through the prevention and relief of distress and suffering by identification of and impeccable assessment and treatment of pain and other problems, physical, psychological and spiritual*" (WHO, 2004). The WHO further emphasized that "*palliative care is an important public health issue…and good quality care towards the end-of-life must be recognized as a basic human right*". In this light, the sustainability of high quality palliative care as well as the promise of a good death for all humanity rests upon health policies and practices that extend beyond the rim of patient care. And this requires a renewed commitment to the promotion of life and mortality, fueled by a public health approach that harnesses the power of an informed, responsible and empathic populace for bolstering the collective strengths of individuals, families and communities in supporting our fellow creatures as well as ourselves who will eventually cross paths with death and loss.

The Imperative of Health Promotion

While 'health promotion' has long been a celebrated strategy for improving population health through policy advocacy and education for illness prevention, 'palliative care' on the other hand emphasizes the care of those whose health have failed and are entering the final stage of illness. By definition, these two terms appear rather contradictory. However, Jan Stjernsward, Director of WHO Collaborating Centre for Palliative Cancer Care, has alluded that in order to ensure sustainable development, there is a critical and urgent need to adopt a 'rational approach' to palliative care, one that transcends the boundaries of institutionalized processes to those that foster public participation (Doyle, Hanks and MacDonald, 1993).

According to the Ottawa Charter, the first international agreement issued by the World Health Organization to encourage global pursuit of "Health for all", health promotion is defined as *"the process of enabling people to increase control over, and to improve, their health. To reach a state of complete physical, mental and social well-being, an individual or group must be able to identify and to realize aspirations, to satisfy needs, and to change or cope with the environment. Health is therefore, seen as a resource for everyday life, not the objective of living. Health is a positive concept emphasizing social and personal resources, as well as physical capacities. Therefore, health promotion is not just the responsibility of the health sector, but goes beyond healthy life-styles to well-being"* (WHO, 1996).

Intrinsically, health promotion requires advocacy, empowerment and mediation so that individuals, families and communities can achieve their fullest health potential within a safe, stable and impartial ecosystem as responsible citizens. The Ottawa Charter further includes five major action statements for realizing the goals of health promotion: (1) build healthy public policy that support health; (2) create supportive environments; (3) strengthen community action; (4) develop personal skills; and (5) reorient health services. In sum, social participation, civil responsibility and informed citizenry form the bedrocks of health promotion (Spoel, Harris and Henwood, 2014). As such, the success of health promoting strategies depends not only upon policy advocacy and public education, but also the recognition that the state of wellbeing is much more than a physical affair, one that required the careful considerations of its social, cultural and environmental characteristics and manifestations.

The Integration of Health Promoting Palliative Care

The aspirations of health promotion can clearly provide the social science and public health perspectives that palliative care greatly needs in order to realize the ideal of quality palliative care for all. As proposed by Community Health Professor Allan Kellehear, the social concepts of health promotion for enhancing individual livelihoods, via relational, environmental and community-based strategies, can first assist in identifying individual and family strengths, establishing social support networks, and guiding individualized regime of health management during the early-stages of terminal illnesses (Kellehear, 1999).

Second, the education and information emphasis of health promotion, which enables people to achieve well-being via making healthy choices, can play an equally important role for helping individuals and families to become more knowledgeable about the illness that they face, consequently empowering them to make informed decisions of care and treatments for maintaining high quality of life at the end of life.

Third, the participatory approach of health promotion can become the impetus for palliative care to cultivate greater involvement in the governance of mortality among every member of society. Sharing, education and learning of illness and death must not be limited to professional caregivers or those who are terminally-ill, but for all persons because death is a common experience shared by all humanity.

Fourth, the structural approach of health promotion for developing policies that are conducive to health and well-being can be adopted in palliative care, serving as a framework to promote public discourse for raising awareness while eliminating the taboos and stigmas of mortality that marginalize the experience of death, dying and bereavement.

Essentially, Health Promoting Palliative Care (HPPC) encourages the development of public policies that support the health of individuals living with life-threatening illnesses; inspire the creation of caring and compassionate environments; strengthen personal skills and social participation; as well as promote the reorientation of health and palliative care services to become more accessible, sustainable and beneficial to those who require them now, and imminently in the future (Kellehear, 1999; 2005). As such, HPPC translate the hospice ideals of 'total pain' and 'whole person care' into much broad public health languages and practices that focus not only on palliation, but also prevention, harm reduction, community action, policy advocacy, research and education.

The Necessity for Life and Death Education

Advocacy that leads to effective policy change must be supported and informed by community engagement and root cause analysis that identify and elicit the needs and voices of all members of society, with a sensitivity that recognizes the assumptions, positions, references, values and beliefs of local cultures. The success of advocacy therefore begins with the introductory work of promoting public discourses through formal and informal education, particularly on the concepts of death, dying, hospice and palliative care (Meier and Beresford, 2007).

Evidence-based life and death education that focuses not only on knowledge and skill transferred, but also on developing one's social-emotional competence and character, then becomes the impetus for enhancing active social participation in mortality. Learning and sharing through experiential and affective education in turn create communal platforms for all societal members to reflect and assess their own perceived needs and wishes at life's end, develop strategies to address them, ultimately leading to greater personal change and community support (Ho and Chan, 2001). Effectively, life and death education serves to build an informed and responsible citizenry, strengthen social capacity and human capital in the management and governance of death and loss, and lay the critical foundation for a basic human right to palliative care.

Over the past two decades, increasing efforts have been placed on implementation of death education programmes in both primary and secondary schools in the West; however, only a minority of the hundreds of millions of children actually receives them (Dennis, 2009). While one may expect that tertiary students get more exposure to the topics of mortality, a survey of 161 colleges and universities in the US found that only 20% offered a course on death, dying and bereavement (Eckerd, 2009). More troubling is the fact that there is inadequate attention given to the learning of death and dying in medical and nursing curricula among most developed countries, as research from the from the past decade have shown that full-course electives are only taken by a fourth of all medical and nursing students in the US and Canada (Dickinson, 1996), while the average medical student in the UK only received 6 hours of life and death-related instructions in a 5 year curriculum (Doyle, 1991). When healthcare providers lack the education to understanding the intricate facets of mortality, as well as the emotional capacity to face the deep emotions of grief and loss, it is difficult to imagine that patients and families can truly be cared for compassionately and with dignity at the end-of-life (Ho, Chan, Leung *et al.*, 2013; Ho, Leung, Tse *et al.*, 2013; Ho, Dai, Lam *et al.*, 2015; Ho, Luk, Chan *et al.*, 2015).

Encouragingly, these disappointing trends of life and death education have taken a turn for the better in very recent years, in both the East and the West. For example, the Harvard Medical School, and the School of Medical Education of King's College of London of the West, as well as the Faculty of Medicine of the University of Hong Kong (HKU), and the new Lee Kong Chian School of Medicine of Nanyang Technological University Singapore (NTU) of the East, have all placed a renewed emphasis in developing and advancing their education and training in Medical Humanities and Mindful Medicine. These programmes, which can now be found in most major medical training institutions across the globe, aspire not only to provide students with a more holistic understanding of the experiences of illness and death, but also to equip students with the science and social skill to practice medicine for the good of humanity, so that they will flourish into *"doctors that you and I would like to be caring for us"* (LKCMedicine, Nanyang Technological University, 2016).

Apart from the training of medical professionals, many universities around the world have also begun to establish a comprehensive undergraduate course on Thanatology; for example, we have developed the course, "The Last Dance: Psycho-Socio-Cultural Perspectives on Death, Dying and Bereavement" at the School of Humanities and Social Sciences at NTU in 2016, which has now become one of the most popular and most demanded seminar course in psychology. My team has also developed a similar course at HKU and it has been receiving the highest student reviews with overwhelming popularity since 2010 (Ho, 2016). Such progress is evident of an ever growing academic and social consciousness that recognizes the important roles that life and death education play in suicide and violence prevention; in correcting the distorted images that glorify or trivialize death; in helping youth and young adults to attain a better understanding of life and mortality, which would ultimately provide them with greater awareness and clarity to recognize and appreciate the finiteness of life, to prioritize goals, to find meaning, as well as to actualize their full potential within the limitless boundaries of being alive.

The Way Forward

As eloquently put by Herman Feifel, founder of Thanatology and pioneer of the modern death awareness movement, "*just as it is belated to start reading sex manuals on the marriage bed, it is rather tardy to begin developing a philosophy of life and death when one is terminally ill or newly bereaved*" (Feifel, 1990). Thus, to resolve the complexity of mortality, we must move beyond our seemingly fruitless pursuit for eternal life (*at least before the promise of Singularity is fulfilled and before we all turn immortal through intelligent machines*), to become informed, responsible, and empathetic citizens who have the knowledge and capacity in facing and managing our own death as well as those of our families, friends and neighbors. A good death can only be achieved through a caring and compassionate community built through advocacy, research and education efforts that aspire towards public health palliative care. In essence, mortality must be recognized not only as a medical and individual issue, but also as a social and collective issue that bonds, connects and unites all humanity.

References

Barley, H. (1995). *Dancing on the Grave*. London: John Murray.

Becker, E. (1973). *The Denial of Death.* New York, NY: Simon & Schuster.

Conway, S. (Ed.) (2012). Governing Death and Loss: Empowerment, involvement and participation. Oxford, UK: Oxford University Press.

Doyle, D. (1991). Palliative care education and training in the United Kingdom: A review. *Death Studies* ***15***, 95–103.

Doyle, D., Hanks, C. W. C., & MacDonald, N. (Eds.). (1993). *Oxford Textbook of Palliative Medicine.* Oxford: Oxford University Press.

Dennis, D., (2009). The past, present, and future of death education. In D. Dennis (Ed.), *Living, Dying, Grieving.* Burlington, MA: Jones & Bartlett Learning.

Dickinson, G. E., Mermann, A. C. (1996). Death education in U.S. medical schools, 1975–1995. *Academic Medicine* ***71***, 1348–1349.

Eckerd, L. M. (2009). Death and dying course offering in psychology: a survey of nine Midwestern states. *Death Studies* ***33***(8), 762–770.

Engel, G. L. (1961). *Is grief a disease? A challenge for medical research.* Psychosomatic Medicine **23**(1), 18–22.

Feifel, H. (1990). Psychology and death: Meaningful rediscovery. *American Psychologist* ***45***, 537–543.

Foucault, M. (1973). *The Birth of the Clinic.* London, UK: Tavistock.

Kellehear, A. (1999). *Health Promoting Palliative Care.* Oxford: Oxford University Press.

Kellehear, A. (2005). *Compassionate Cities: Public Health and End-of-Life Care.* London: Routledge.

Kubler-Ross, R. (1970). *On Death and Dying.* London, UK: Tavistock.

Ham, C. (1994). *Health Policy in Britain.* London, England: MacMillan Press.

Ho, A. H. Y. (2016). *Health Promoting Palliative Care through Higher Education Reform: Development and Evaluation of a New Humanities Course in Thanatology* (Unpublished doctoral dissertation). University of Nottingham, UK.

Ho, A. H. Y., & Chan, C. L. W. (2011). Liberating bereaved persons from the oppression of death and loss in Chinese societies: examples of the public health approaches. In S. Conway (ed.) *Governing Death and Loss: Empowerment, Involvement and Participation,* pp. 119–128. UK: Oxford University Press.

Ho, A. H. Y., Chan, C. L. W., Leung, P. P. Y., Chochinov, H. M., Neimeyer, R. A., Pang, S. M. C., & Tse, D. M. W. (2013). Living and Dying with Dignity in Chinese Society: Perspectives of Older Palliative Care Patients in Hong Kong. *Age and Ageing* ***42***(4), 455–461.

Ho, A. H. Y., Dai, A. A. N., Lam, S. H., Wong, S. W. P., Tsui, A. L. M., Tang, J. C. S., & Lou, V. W. Q. (2015). Development and Pilot evaluation of a novel dignity-conserving end-of-life (EoL) care model for nursing homes in Chinese societies. *The Gerontologist,* DOI: 10.1093/geront/gnv037.

Ho, A. H. Y., Leung, P. P. Y., Tse, D. M. W., Pang, S. M. C., Chochinov, H. M., Neimeyer, R. A. & Chan, C. L. W. (2013). Dignity amidst liminality: Suffering within healing among Chinese terminal cancer patients. *Death Studies* ***37***(10), 953–970.

Ho, A. H. Y., Luk, J. K. H., Chan, F. H. W., Ng, W. C., Kowk, C. K. K., Yuen, J. H. L., Tam, M. Y. J., Kan, W. S., & Chan, C. L. W. (2015). Dignified palliative care in long-term care settings: An interpretive-systemic framework of end-of-life integrated care pathway for terminally-ill Chinese older adults. *American Journal of Hospice and Palliative Medicine,* DOI: 10.1177/1049909114565789.

Illich, I. (1976). *Medical Nemesis: The Exploration of Health.* New York, NY: Pantheon Books.

Lee Kong Chian Medicine, Nanyang Technological University (2016). *Ethos of Education. Retrieved from: http://www.lkcmedicine.ntu.edu.sg/aboutus/Pages/VisionMissionandValues.aspx.*

Meier, D., & Beresford, L. (2007). Advocacy is essential to palliative care's future development. *Journal of Palliative Medicine* ***10***, 840–844.

O'Gorman, S. M. (1998). Death and dying in contemporary society: An evaluation of current attitudes and the rituals associated with death and dying and their relevance to recent understanding of health and healing. *Journal of Advanced Nursing* ***24***, 1127–1135.

Ray Kurzeil (2005). *The Singularity is Near.* New York: Penguin Group.

Parsons, T. (1963). Death in American society: A brief working paper. *American Behavioral Scientist* **6**, 61–65.

Saunders, C. (1967). St. Christopher's Hospice. N*ursing Times* ***28***, 988–999.

Shryock, R. N. (1947). *The Development of Modern Medicine. An Interpretation of Social and Scientific Factors Involved* (2nd Ed). New York, NY: Knopf.

Spoel, P., Harris, R., & Henwood, F. (2014). Rhetorics of health citizenship: Exploring vernacular critiques of government's role in supporting healthy living. *Journal of Medical Humanities* ***35***, 131–147.

Sweeting, H. N., & Gilhooley, L. M. (1992). Doctor, am I dead? A review of social death in modern societies. *Omega: Journal of Death and Dying* ***24***(2), 251–269.

World Health Organization. (1996). The Ottawa Charter for Health Promotion. Geneva. Switzerland: WHO.

World Health Organization. (2004). *The Solid Facts: Palliative Care.* Geneva, Switzerland: WHO.

10 Is Consciousness a Riddle Wrapped in a Mystery inside an Enigma? Mysterianism and Beyond

Roger Vergauwen

Katholieke Universiteit Leuven,
Institute of Philosophy,
Center for Logic and Analytic Philosophy,
Kardinaal Mercierplein 2, 3000 Leuven, Belgium
roger.vergauwen@kuleuven.be

Introduction

The philosopher D. Dennett is credited with coining three different 'stances' all useful in predicting the behaviour of certain systems and objects [Dennett, 1987].

In the *Design Stance* one predicts the behaviour of a system by assuming that it has a certain design, that it is composed of certain elements with certain functions and that it will behave as it is designed to behave under certain circumstances. In so doing the design stance can safely ignore details of the physical implementation of the various imputed functions.

In the *Physical Stance* one predicts the behaviour of physical systems by exploiting information about the physical constituents of the system and the laws of physics.

And finally there is the *Intentional Stance* in which the systems whose behaviour one wants to predict are treated as rational agents. They are attributed the beliefs and desires they ought to have given their place in the world and their purpose, and subsequently one predicts that they will act to further their goals in the light of their beliefs. As such these different stances present some kind of cumulative hierarchy in which one level builds upon the other thus presenting a picture of intertwined relations that together explain the behaviour of complex systems such as also the human being.

Some philosophers have argued for an additional stance beyond the three that Dennett outlined. They call it the *Phenomenal Stance* [Robbins and Jack, 2006]. Here one argues about the attribution of consciousness, emotions and inner experience to a mind. The problem of the so-called *Explanatory Gap* considered as the *Hard Problem of Consciousness* to some illustrates the tendency of people to see *Phenomenal Experience* as different from physical processes [Chalmers, 1995].

This paper consists of five parts. The first and second parts will show how in contemporary philosophy of mind and consciousness the physical stance (as an example of a naturalistic approach to consciousness) is the overarching paradigm. Here, we will concentrate on the so-called problem of *Qualia* – with a digression on Language – more specifically on the question of their existence and their neurobiological explanation.

In the third part *Mysterianist Theories of Mind and Consciousness* will be discussed. Strangely enough, these theories themselves claim to be naturalistic and belong thus to the physical stance, but it will be shown that the naturalism proposed is self-contradictory and misguided, though it may help to pave the way for an approach which one might consider to belong to the Phenomenal Stance though it does not suffer from the defects that can be attributed to Mysterianism and is fully compatible with contemporary neuro-biological approaches. This will be discussed in a fourth part, which will concentrate on such concepts as embodied information and certain logical or – rather – metalogical properties that this information may possess, thereby elucidating the central concept of the (conscious) *Self as a Quale*.

In a final, concluding, part it will be shown how a transcultural approach combined with empirical research can contribute to a deeper understanding of the phenomenon of consciousness. Specifically, philosophical views in East and West alike have been formulated with respect to the aforementioned central concept of the Self. The Buddhist tradition of the so-called *Non-Self Theories* will be used to illustrate this point.

Qualia, Linguistics and Science

In recent discussions in the Philosophy of Mind the nature of phenomenal states or qualia – also called 'raw feels', 'conscious sensations', or the feel of *'what it is like to be'* – and of consciousness in general have been an important focus of research. Qualia, then, are (first order) properties of mental states such as e.g. 'seeing red', 'feeling pain' and the concept is sometimes used more broadly to indicate conscious experience in general. Explaining these qualia has been called 'the hard problem of consciousness': David Chalmers, e.g., writes: "If any problem qualifies as *the* problem of consciousness, it is this one. In this central sense of 'consciousness', an organism is conscious if there is something it is like to be that organism, and a mental state is conscious if there is something it is like to be in that state. Sometimes terms such as 'phenomenal consciousness' and Qualia are used here" [Chalmers 1995, p. 201].

Functionalists hold that mental states, qualia, and cognitive states in general can be viewed as the functional states of a machine or, rather, of a Turing-machine. In this view, the explanation of cognitive functions has to be done in terms of a causal-functional description of these functions. So e.g. a typical functional explanation of 'pain' would imply that pain is a functional state and as such, therefore, functions as the detection of tissue-damage. Of course, such a causal-functional state or role may cause the production of a certain behaviour or of another functional state which is the result of the first state. In functionalism, a mental state is defined in terms of three elements which are causally related: the input – the stimulation which causes the mental state – the causal interaction with other mental states, and the output which is behavioural. In this sense mental states are defined by means of a job description. Reductive explanations in science usually work this way. It is, e.g., known that organisms are able to transmit hereditary information. This was known even before the gene was discovered. Subsequent scientific investigations showed that in fact DNA was responsible for this transmission and that therefore did the job that was required [Kim 1998, p. 10].

It is within such a functionalist framework that some have argued that Chomsky's approach, who considers linguistics to be part of cognitive psychology, is misguided. Michael Devitt and Kim Sterelny [Devitt and Sterelny, 1989] have presented an argument – dubbed the *Martian Argument* by Stephen Laurence – intended to show why this is so. Linguistics, according to Chomsky, deals with human knowledge and understanding of language, linguistic competence, and is therefore concerned with questions about the cognitive skills of human beings and thus in the end is ultimately about the specific human neural setup. The psychological mechanisms for language acquisition are instantiated into the mind/brains of the human language users.

Since grammars are about such instantiations, the instantiation of English grammar in humans is indeed English according to this conception. This we may call the *Competence Thesis*, the thesis that grammars are about the human language competence. The Martian argument, now, runs as follows. Let us assume that Martians, whose psycholinguistic processes *ex hypothesi* differ from human ones nevertheless manage to produce a set of sentences that are extensionally equivalent to the set of sentences in human English. This implies that the sentences that are grammatical in Martian English are also grammatical in regular English.

However, since by hypothesis Martians have a different neural organization they really have a different language competence and now the question arises whether they should count as speaking English? On an account of what it is to speak English the Martian speakers should indeed count as speaking English. On the level of linguistic symbols everything they say is indistinguishable from us and they also seem to be able to communicate via a seemingly shared language. They are, therefore, on the face of it, competent in English. We can, then, nevertheless study the shared language that we both use on the linguistic level without having to appeal to differences in competence.

"According to the transformationalists, English competence consists in internalizing a grammar. They go further: all English speakers have internalized near enough the one grammar; competence has a uniform structure across the linguistic community. Even if this is so, it is not necessarily so. Many other grammars could agree on the meaning-relevant structures they assign to the sentences of English. Suppose that Martians became competent in English by internalizing one of these other grammars. The theory of Martian competence would have to be different from the theory of ours. Yet the theory of symbols would be the same, for it would still be English that they spoke. Returning to earth, it would not matter a lot to the theory of symbols if competence among actual English speakers was entirely idiosyncratic" [Devitt and Sterelny 1989, p. 514]. This argument has caused a lot of discussion which we do not want to go into here but we want to maintain that this functionalist approach, which is in fact nothing but a variant of the Turing test, neglects an hitherto not enough noticed fact, namely that 'there is something it is like to use (speak and understand) a (specific) language' which in turn means that in fact the ability to use a language turns out to be some kind of a quale. Moreover, functionalism at best does not believe that qualia can be fully functionalized and because of the Supervenience Principle, according to Kim and others, in combination with certain intuitively plausible assumptions (causal exclusion principles) it implies a kind of epiphenomenalism, the view that every mental event is caused by a physical event in the brain but that mental events have no causal powers of their own.

They are powerless to cause anything else, not even other mental events and are therefore almost literally 'non-existent'.

In our view language and consciousness are intimately related and have a 'phenomenal' ('qualia-like') aspect. A further investigation into the nature of these qualia may, therefore, then reveal something of the true nature of the mental state and of language.

Neuroscientists and philosophers alike have been stressing the importance of the phenomenal aspect of consciousness and this also transpires in the way scientists look upon the phenomenal aspect of consciousness.

Neurobiology and Qualia

As an example [Vergauwen 2010, pp. 1258-1260], the neurobiological model proposed by Gerald Edelman, more specifically, his theory of *Neuronal Group Selection* where he uses the concept of a *Dynamic Core* could be considered. Edelman explicitly aims at constructing a naturalized theory of consciousness, in which properties such as intentionality – the fact that conscious mental states are characterized by 'aboutness' – and qualia – the subjective 'raw feels' – are accounted for in a neural framework. He begins by stressing that, though it is sometimes claimed that any attempt to reduce phenomenal or subjective experience (qualia) to neural activities leads to an explanatory gap which constitutes 'the hard problem of consciousness', this need not be a problem because in a certain sense a reduction is possible: "the neural systems underlying consciousness arose to enable high-order discriminations in a multidimensional space of signals (and) qualia are those discriminations. Differences in qualia correlate with differences in the neural structure and the dynamics that underlie them... and I have stressed that it is the distinction among the entire set of experienced qualia that allow the specific defining property of each quale to appear" [Edelman 2003, p. 5521].

However, a scientific account of the individual experiences of these qualia is not to be expected since: "a scientific theory cannot presume to replicate the experience that it describes or explains: a theory to account for a hurricane is not a hurricane. A third-person description by a theorist of the qualia associated with wine tasting can, for example, take detailed account of the reported personal experiences of that theorist and his human subjects. It cannot, however, directly convey or induce qualia by description: to experience the discriminations of an individual it is necessary to be that individual" [Edelman 2003, p. 2251]. In other words simulation is not duplication.

Consciousness, in this view, arises from re-entrant interactions among neural populations and the causal activity is produced by the dynamic core; so, the qualia emerging from this core are caused by it, but, according to Edelman this does not necessarily lead to epiphenomenalism because these emerging qualia are informational structures even if they are not causal and it may sometimes be useful to talk about these qualitative informational states 'as-if' they are causal depending on the level of description. This does not, however, imply epiphenomenalism, since "There is, however, no need to conclude that C [qualia] is therefore meaningless and unnecessary. C states [qualia-states] are informational even if not causal. C states are the discriminations entailed by causal transactions among C [neural states]" [Edelman 2003, p. 5523]. The qualia, then, are the reflections of the permanent causal interactions in the (complex) dynamic core, but are themselves not causally active: "underlying each quale are distinct neuroanatomical structures and neural dynamics that together account for the specific and distinctive phenomenal property of that quale" [Edelman 2003, p. 5523].

As for the phenomenal experience of the quale itself the theory holds that it is no problem – and that therefore the 'hard problem' and the problem of the 'explanatory gap' are ill posed – because the need for a phenotype experiencing and giving rise to the qualia is no hindrance for a scientific theory of consciousness and, moreover, "if the phenomenal part of conscious experience that constitutes its entailed distinctions is irreducible, so is the fact that physics has not explained why there is something rather than nothing" [Edelman 2003, p. 5524].

A main tenet of Edelman's thesis is the concept of re-entrant signalling between neuronal groups. He defines re-entry as the ongoing recursive dynamic interchange of signals that occurs in parallel between brain maps, and which continuously interrelates these maps to each other in time and space. Re-entry depends for its operations on the intricate networks of massively parallel reciprocal connections within and between neuronal groups, which arise through processes of developmental and experiential selection. Edelman describes re-entry as a form of ongoing higher-order selection that appears to be unique to animal brains and concludes that "there is no other object in the known universe so completely distinguished by re-entrant circuitry as the human brain" [Edelman and Tononi 2000,

p. 49]. So, in fact the human brain is a massively recursive machine and therefore also computable.[1]

It should, then, come as no surprise that in this view human language inherits this recursion. Indeed, in a *Science* article Hauser, Chomsky and Fitch [Hauser *et al.,* 2002] have suggested that recursion is a basic characteristic that distinguishes human language from all other forms of animal communication and that, indeed, human consciousness itself is characterized by recursiveness [Corballis, 2011].

However, at the very heart of the discussion still is the nature of qualia and of consciousness itself within a naturalistic paradigm [Manzotti, R. and Moderato P., 2010]. If we assume that qualia can be causally active (be it as informational states) they are in principle amenable to scientific investigation and to some kind of naturalistic reduction. Some philosophers, among which Colin McGinn, have argued that naturalism can be combined with a view that leaves consciousness somehow a 'mystery' in the sense that the hard problem of consciousness cannot be resolved by human beings thus presenting a view that is a variant of non-reductive physicalism.

Mysterianism: McGinn's Answer to the Mind-Body Problem[2]

The problem of consciousness has been generally recognized as the hard problem of the mind-body problem. Dualism, materialism, idealism, have all produced their own answers and solutions, but the problem and the mystery remain. McGinn summarizes the situation as follows: "how is it possible for conscious states to depend upon brain states? How can technicolour phenomenology arise from soggy grey matter? What makes the bodily organ we call the brain so radically different from other bodily organs, say the kidneys – the body parts without a trace of consciousness? How could the aggregation of millions of insentient neurons generate subjective awareness? We know that brains are the *de facto* causal basis of consciousness, but we have, it seems, no understanding whatever of how this can be so. It strikes us as miraculous, eerie, even faintly comic. Somehow, we feel, the water of the physical brain is turned into the wine of consciousness, but we draw a total blank on the nature of this conversion" [McGinn 1989, pp. 349]. Any proposed solution to the mind-body problem should, in McGinn's view, start from

[1] The consequences of this view will be explored in part 4.
[2] See also: [Vergauwen, 2014]

what he calls 'Transcendental Naturalism' and the conceptual and cognitive 'closure' of human beings.

Transcendental naturalism

McGinn's solution to the mind-body problem, which has been dubbed *Mysterianism,* because it relies on the idea of a mystery being a question that happens to fall outside of a given creature's cognitive space [McGinn 1993, p. 3], starts from what he calls transcendental naturalism. According to transcendental naturalism [McGinn 1993, pp. 3-8] about a certain question Q with respect to a certain being B, it may be the case that the answer to that question is beyond the (cognitive) capacities of such a being. That is, the answer to a certain question may be epistemically inaccessible to a certain being. This is what he calls cognitive closure.

McGinn maintains that consciousness is a natural phenomenon, arising from the organizations of matter [McGinn 1989, p. 353], but at the same time advocates epistemic irreducibility, being the view that holds that there is no explanation of consciousness available to us because of the cognitive closure of the human mind. Summarizing:

1a. There exists a property P, which is instantiated in the brain, and which is the causal basis of consciousness.
1b. Identifying this property can be done in basically two different ways, viz. direct investigation through introspection or empirical study of the brain.
1c. Direct investigation through introspection cannot identify P.
1d. Empirical study of the brain cannot identify P.
1e. Therefore, P cannot be identified.

Conceptual and cognitive closure

That direct investigation through introspection cannot be used to identify the required property seems evident. It is of course true that we have immediate access to our own consciousness and its properties, but this does not imply that the required property could be found in this way because by itself this introspection does not reveal the nature of P. Introspection, McGinn argues, reveals our experience to us but it does not reveal to us how conscious states depend upon brain states. An analysis of the concept of consciousness by means of some procedure of conceptual analysis will not do either because by such an analysis we will not be able to see how consciousness depends upon the brain any more than we could solve the problem of how life depends upon physical properties by reflecting on the concept of *life.* Therefore, in as far as introspection could be used as a tool to construct concepts with respect to the nature of P, it is conceptually closed with respect to P.

But, according to McGinn, an empirical investigation of the brain cannot be of help either if we want to understand the nature of P. He wants to argue that P is also perceptually closed to us: "the argument for perceptual closure starts from the thought that nothing we can imagine perceiving in the brain would ever convince us that we have located the intelligible nexus we seek. No matter what recondite property we could see to be instantiated in the brain we would always be baffled about how it could give rise to consciousness... Inference to the best explanation of purely physical data will never take us outside the realm of the physical, forcing us to introduce concepts of consciousness" [McGinn 1989, pp. 357-358]. Our senses are geared towards a representation of the spatial world and do therefore represent things as essentially existing in space and therefore with spatial properties [McGinn 1989, p. 363 n21]. Since consciousness is not spatially defined, it falls outside the realm of our observational capacities and it cannot be grasped by our spatially-oriented senses. It is, then, because the empirical property that is supposed to provide the causal nexus between the brain and the mind is *noumenal* with respect to our senses that we will never be able to provide an answer to the mind-body problem.

Contrary to what one might expect, McGinn does not think that there is no scientific solution to the mind-body problem. In his view, consciousness has an explanation "in a certain science, but this science is inaccessible to us as a matter of principle" [McGinn 1989, p. 362]. Whatever else this science may be like, it is clear that at least one principle will probably have it be upheld which is the principle of causality already well defined by Hume: "...All arguments concerning existence are founded on the relation of cause and effect; that our knowledge of that relation is entirely from experience; and all of experimental conclusions proceed upon the supposition that the future will be conformable to the past" [Hume 1777, pp. 36-37]. Even if McGinn has a very different science in mind, causality in some sense will have to be present there and the mind-brain relation can, therefore, not be totally a priori.

Science, effective decidability and truth

It can be shown that it is McGinn's view of the interpretation of the semantics of his own Transcendental Naturalism that is a further basis for his mysterianism, since it crucially makes use of the concept of *recognition-transcendent truth-conditions.* This position, then, may be summarized as follows [McGinn 1989, pp. 352-362]:

2a. There exists a property, P, instantiated by the brain, in virtue of which the brain is the basis of consciousness. In particular, P provides the causal basis of consciousness.

2b. P is the spatial causal basis of the non-spatial (consciousness).

2c. We are (probably absolutely) cognitively closed to P or to a theory which contains P.

2d. P has a full and non-mysterious explanation in a certain science that is inaccessible to us as a matter of principle.

(2d) indicates that the problem involved is also an epistemological one, in the sense that we are not required to abandon our materialist intuitions to acknowledge a mysterious non-material mind. So, the mystery is not metaphysical. However, at the same time (2a) is a proposition which, because of (2c-d), has recognition-transcendent truth-conditions (for human beings). It is not effectively decidable from our perspective and our science. In McGinn's view, the proposition (2a) is nevertheless also true and even effectively decided (2d).

But why does McGinn think that (2a) is true? The answer is surprisingly simple, albeit not unproblematic: "the philosophical problem about consciousness and the brain arises from a sense that we are compelled to accept that nature contains miracles – as if the merely metallic lamp of the brain could really spirit into existence the Djin of consciousness. But we do not need to accept this: we can rest secure in the knowledge that some (unknowable) property of the brain makes everything fall into place. What creates the philosophical puzzlement is the assumption that the problem must somehow be scientific but that any science *we* can come up with will represent things as utterly miraculous" [McGinn 1989, p. 362]. So, in fact, it is his (belief in) *naturalism* which forces McGinn to accept the truth of (2a). (2a) is effectively decidable (and even effectively decided), according to McGinn, but only in a science that is inaccessible to us, since we are cognitively closed to it. That is why its truth-conditions are in fact recognition-transcendent (for us) and therefore also not effectively decidable.

It is McGinn's conviction that, since our conceptual and scientific frameworks are thoroughly permeated by concepts that are essentially spatial, these concepts are unsuitable to study the nature of consciousness, which is non-spatial. Such a study would require 'leaving behind' the spatial framework of our thinking and that would mean losing the ability to distinguish among things, since we use spatial resources to identify things as particulars: "understanding consciousness as it really is would require us to jettison the spatial skeleton of our thought – leaving us with no propositions and so nothing with which to think" [Rowlands 2010, p. 341].

However, in order for (2d) to be necessarily true, it should be true in all possible worlds that are accessible from our world [Gamut 1991, p. 22], such is the logical semantics of modal propositions. What McGinn is describing in (2d) is a proposition which, in order for it to be true, it should be true in a world that is in principle inaccessible from our world, since that is what the proposition says, which makes it difficult to believe that (2d) is a proposition that is necessarily true. It would seem, then, that (2d) cannot be necessarily true and might, therefore, be false. So, if (2d) is necessarily true, it might be false, which is a contradiction. Therefore (2d) is not necessarily true, McGinn's speculations notwithstanding. Alternatively, one might also say that naturalism and realism are false, since the combination of naturalism and realism forces McGinn to say that (2d) is necessarily true. We might say that what McGinn is trying to establish is that some propositions have what we could call *absolutely experience-transcending truth-conditions.* The problem is the combination of naturalism, effective decidability, absolutely experience-transcending truth-conditions and the concept of cognitive closure. From our discussion it appears that such a combination is incoherent.

Consciousness, Information and Incompleteness

Even though mysterianism as defended by McGinn is questionable and self-refuting, there does indeed seem to be an explanatory gap in our understanding of consciousness as McGinn rightly indicates and it has to do with the fact that conscious states are phenomenal states. In other words, conscious states are qualitative in character and that is also why the problem of consciousness is sometimes identified with the problem of qualia. On the face of it and up to a certain extent, this explanatory gap is a consequence of an asymmetry between the third- and first-person perspective: "due to this asymmetry, we have to expect such a 'phenomenal difference' even if we observe one and the same process from either perspective, and we can explain why this is so" [Pauen 1998, p. 204]. But maybe something else is also to be considered, which is related to the nature of the information processed by the brain.

Consciousness and information

The theory of consciousness we want to present here is to a certain extent tributary to David Chalmers' so-called 'Double-Aspect theory of Information': his hypothesis is that information has two fundamental aspects, a physical one and an experiential or phenomenal one, and that, furthermore, phenomenal consciousness by virtue of its status is one aspect of information where the other aspect is found embodied in physical processing. Physical information is, as embodied information, then, "a difference that makes a difference": "The basic principle that I suggest centrally involves the notion of *information.* I understand information in more or less the sense of Shannon (1948). Where there is information, there are *information states* embedded in an *information space.* An information space has a basic structure of difference relations between its elements, characterizing the ways in which different elements in a space are similar or different, possibly in complex ways. An information space is an abstract object, but following Shannon we can see information as *physically embodied* when there is a space of distinct physical states, the differences between which can be transmitted down some causal pathway. The states that are transmitted can be seen as themselves constituting an information space. To borrow a phrase from Bateson (1972), physical information is *a difference that makes a difference*" [Chalmers 1995, p. 216].

What Chalmers is claiming is that phenomenal properties (qualia) constitute the internal aspect of information. This is what he calls the Double-Aspect Theory of information, and it is one of a number of psychophysical principles, principles connecting the properties of physical processes to the properties of experience.

Chalmers notes that there are certain structural analogies between the physical and the phenomenal aspects of information: "there is a direct isomorphism between certain physically embodied information spaces and certain phenomenal (or experiential) information spaces... That is, we can find the same abstract information space embedded in physical processing and in conscious experience" [Chalmers 1995, p. 21]. Inevitably, at this moment questions of computability of this kind of information show up.

Consciousness and computability

One of the limits on the computability of a system is that it may be undecidable in a strict logical sense as is proven in Gödel's famous

Incompleteness Theorems. Roger Penrose, for one, has suggested how quantum mechanics may help to explain how the human mind goes beyond Turing Computability [Penrose, 1994, 2013]. He does not talk explicitly about qualia but, rather, about mathematical creativity and uses Gödel's Incompleteness Theorems to show how human beings can 'see' the truth of certain mathematical propositions even though within an axiomatic system these propositions are undecidable, i.e. neither the propositions themselves nor their negations can be proven. This makes the system *incomplete.* Though one may say here, as Chalmers does, that this non-algorithmic (non-computable) processing is another example of an 'extra ingredient' which may tell us something about the physical role that conscious experience plays but not how it arises, the point I want to raise here is a different one.

If Chalmers is right in saying that phenomenal properties constitute the internal aspect of information, then a *metalogical property such as incompleteness* which is definitely a property of (complex) formalized mathematical systems is also a property of the information the system contains. Mental states and natural language are usually characterized as being 'intentional'. Intentionality or 'aboutness' is a term coined by the Austrian philosopher Franz Brentano which points towards the directedness upon the world of mental states in general and of language in particular, their content, or their (possibly non-existing) reference.

In view of the theory presented here we suggest that there is a close relationship between intentionality, logical incompleteness and consciousness. If a system is logically incomplete it means that it has non-isomorphic models, also called *non-standard models,* which is for instance the case with the models of formalized arithmetic in Gödel's incompleteness theorems. This comes down to the fact that the information in the axioms of the theory is in a sense insufficient to uniquely determine what they are 'about'. Incompleteness may, then, be seen as a logical analogue of intentionality in the following sense.

In the Correspondence Theory of Meaning and Truth which states that the truth or falsity of a proposition is determined by how it relates to the world and whether it accurately describes it – 'corresponds with' – that world [Hannah and Harrison, 2004] the property of truth expresses the 'aboutness' of propositions in the sense that true propositions are 'true of' or 'about' true states of affairs. The property of truth, therefore, expresses the 'reference-relation' for such propositions. If truth is non-computable or non-algorithmic, then so is intentionality. If Penrose is right, human beings are able to 'see' the truth of certain mathematical statements and are therefore able to perform non-computable operations which Penrose thinks are a consequence of non-computable elements in the physical laws which the brain exploits when it performs this task. One need not agree with Penrose's idea of performing non-computable tasks to see that the general phenomenon of incompleteness might epistemologically indicate that the 'aboutness' is a consequence of a tension between the inside ('information') of the system and the outside of the world – which might as a felt distinction be called *The Self* – which is what the information is supposed to be about, a tension which in turn is a consequence of the embodiment of the information processed by the mind. The intentionality of (phenomenal) consciousness and of language might, then, be said to derive from the same source: the incompleteness of the information processed by the brain. If this system would be complete in the logical sense, the system itself would be *categorical* so that all of its models would be isomorphic. But that would at the same time imply that the 'tension' between the information and what it is about would disappear. The feeling of 'aboutness' which we find in (certain) conscious mental states and in language might then, somewhat speculatively, be defined as the reflection of the difference between language and 'the world'.

Assuming that the information processed in conscious states also exhibits this kind of incompleteness, this might, phenomenally be experienced as a 'felt' distinction between the inside of the system (the conscious mind) and the outside world with which the system interacts and therefore create the feeling of subjectivity. In this sense the first-person or subjective point of view (the 'what-is-it-like' or 'phenomenal' point of view) has a logical analogue in the incompleteness of the information processed. This does not exclude that conscious processes are identified with brain processes, but it does suggest that the quest for the nature of consciousness should be pursued on a higher level of information-processing even though certain properties of the brain are causally responsible for consciousness. Such a view may avoid the difficulties and pitfalls that go with McGinn's mysterianism without necessarily leading to a reductionist naturalism.

Conclusion: Consciousness and East-West Self-Imagery

Our reference to Gödel's Incompleteness Theorems and their possible importance for the study of consciousness also has its importance on a broader scientific-cultural level. Indeed, the phenomena Gödel described through the process of *Arithmetization* (thus making mathematics 'talk about itself') indicate that the systems he has in mind allow for self-reference or reflexivity. Recent research concerning experimental and theoretical approaches to conscious processing indicates that the phenomenon of consciousness should not be limited to conscious access but that additional, higher-order concepts of consciousness are also needed.

Some researchers believe that the core consciousness of incoming sensory information requires integrating it with a sense of *self* (the specific subjective point of view of the perceiving organism which is in fact the phenomenal or qualitative view), while others think that a higher-order thought, coding for the very fact that the organism is currently representing a piece of information, is needed for that information to be conscious. It is here that meta-cognition, or the ability to reflect upon thoughts and draw judgements upon them, is often proposed as a crucial ingredient of consciousness [Dehaene and Changeux 2011, p. 218].

To many contemporary philosophers of mind the phenomenon of consciousness requires some kind of self-referentiality or reflexivity which is at least partially responsible for its phenomenal character and for the production of the self. In this tradition, the question whether subjectivity requires a self or subject and whether consciousness is intrinsically reflexive have come to be closely linked. However, at the same time it should be noted that this tradition is tributary to a specific cultural and philosophical point of view. Indeed, we might classify views about the self as falling into several broad types: substantialist, non-substantialist and non-self theories. While non-self theorists deny the existence of a self, substantialist and non-substantialist self theorists affirm its existence but disagree about its nature. Substantialists take the view that the self is a substance in which different properties are located at one time or at different times. Non-substantialist self theorists hold that the self is not a substance standing in relation to a consciousness that is somehow distinct from it, but consider the self as just consciousness itself. The non-self view is hardly known in the West but it has been extensively discussed in the Buddhist tradition. Buddhist philosophy aims at proving that there is no entity that might serve as the referent of 'I' and attempts to explain how the belief that there is such an entity might have come into existence. This is the famous doctrine of the no(n)-self *(anattā/anātman).* However, while some Buddhist philosophers do indeed claim that subjectivity does not require a self or subject, they still hold that consciousness is intrinsically reflexive in order to account for the phenomenal (subjective or 'qualitative') character of conscious states, others – especially within the early

Theravāda school of Buddhism – do in fact not accept the reflexivity of consciousness. From the fact that subjectivity requires a subject or self and from the fact that there is no self, they deduce that consciousness is irreflexive. So, in this sense consciousness is 'ownerless'.

In an intriguing paper, Mark Sideritis [Sideritis, 2013] speculates about the consequences of such a view. After a long and winding argument which includes a discussion of both Buddhist and non-Buddhist Indian 'other-illuminationists' he concludes that mental states have the property of being conscious only extrinsically, through their relations to other states, and are therefore reducible as some kind of cognitive states acting upon other cognitive states. It would follow that if in this respect the fact that we think we are conscious is just a useful way for a certain sort of information-processing system to manage the flow of information, then there is no need for a self to explain the fact that the system self-represents, a view that is strikingly similar to contemporary functionalist views on consciousness and concludes that, if anything, consciousness can only be known indirectly: "Consciousness is, on this view, irreflexive, just like everything else in the universe. No more is consciousness aware of itself than a knife cuts itself or a fingertip touches itself. We can nonetheless be aware not only of a pot, but of our awareness of a pot. This must be achieved through a distinct cognition. But the cognition in question is not a case of reflection or inner perception. It is indirect. This makes it a case of what we would call inference" [Sideritis 2013, p. 324]. Sideritis goes further than this and concludes that, since consciousness cannot be perceived its occurrence cannot be known through inference and that it is therefore as a qualitative phenomenon, strictly speaking, non-existing.

We do not, I think, need to agree with this conclusion in order to draw certain lessons from its premises. Specifically, it seems to be a consequence of the denial of the reflexivity of consciousness and its reduction to mental states monitoring other mental states that it can be described in terms of an inferential cognitive process and thus as a form of meta-cognition or indirect cognition in the way some contemporary brain-researchers have in mind. If there is no self, consciousness can only be known by inference to the best explanation and it becomes irreflexive.

It would seem, then, that the importance one attaches to the self influences the view one has on the nature of consciousness itself. The Buddhist idea of no-self creates a philosophical paradigm which might also have an influence on the way in which consciousness is studied scientifically. It would, therefore, be worthwhile to study the empirical consequences of both East and West approaches (the self-approach and the indirect cognition approach) and in doing so we would have a prime example of a fruitful interaction between neuroscientific and philosophical approaches in East and West.

References

Chalmers, D. (1995) Facing up the Problem of Consciousness, *J. of Consciousness Studies,* 2(3), pp. 200-219.

Corballis, M. C. (2011) *The recursive Mind: The Origins of human Language, Thought, and Civilization*, Princeton University Press.

Dehaene, S. and Changeux, J.-P. (2011) Experimental and Theoretical Approaches to Conscious Processing, *Neuron,* 70, pp. 200-227.

Dennett, D. (1987) *The Intentional Stance,* MIT Press.

Devitt, M. and Sterelny, K. (1989) Linguistics: what's wrong with "the Right View"?, *Philosophical Perspectives,* 3, pp. 498-531.

Edelman, G. (2003) Naturalizing Consciousness. A theoretical Framework, *Proceedings of the National Academy of Sciences,* 100(9), pp. 5520-5524.

Edelman, G. and Tononi, G. (2000) *A Universe of Consciousness: how Matter becomes Imagination*, Basic Books (New York).

Gamut, L. T. F. (1991) *Logic, Language and Meaning: Volume 2. Intensional Logic and Logical Grammar*, University of Chicago Press.

Hannah, P. and Harrison, B. (2004) *Word and World: Practices and the Foundation of Language,* Cambridge University Press.

Hauser, M., Chomsky, N. and Fitch, W.T. (2002) The Faculty of Language: What Is It, who Has It, and How Did It Evolve?, *Science,* 298, pp. 1569-1579.

Hume, D. (1777) *Enquiries concerning the Human Understanding and concerning the Principles of Morals* (Selby-Bigge, L. A. (Ed.)), Clarendon Press.

Kim, J. (1998) *Philosophy of Mind*, Westview Press.

McGinn, C. (1989) Can we solve The Mind-Body Problem?, *Mind,* 392, pp. 349-366.

McGinn, C. (1993) *Problems in Philosophy: The Limits of Enquiry*, Blackwell.

Manzotti R. and Moderato R. (2010) Is Neuroscience adequate as the forthcoming "Mindscience"?, *Behavior and Philosophy,* 38, pp. 1-29.

Pauen, M. (1998) Is there an empirical answer to the explanatory gap problem?, *Consciousness and Cognition,* 7, pp. 202-205.

Penrose, R. (1994) *Shadows of the Mind: A Search for the Missing Science of Consciousness*, Oxford University Press.

Penrose, R. (2013) Foreword, in Zenil, H. (Ed.), *A Computable Universe: Understanding and Exploring Nature as Computation,* pp. xiii-xxxvi, World Scientific.

Robbins, P. and Jack, T. (2006) The Phenomenal Stance, *Philosophical Studies*, 127, pp. 59-85.

Rowlands, M. (2010) Mysterianism, in Velmans, M. and Schneider, S. (Eds.), *The Blackwell Companion to Consciousness,* pp. 335-345, Blackwell.

Sideritis, M. (2013) Buddhas as Zombies: A Buddhist Reduction of Subjectivity, in Sideritis, M., Thompson, E. and Zahavi, D., *Self, No Self?: Perspectives from Analytical, Phenomenological, & Indian Traditions,* pp. 308-331, Oxford University Press.

Vergauwen, R. (2010) Will Science and Consciousness ever Meat? Complexity, Symmetry and Qualia, *Symmetry,* 2, pp. 1250-1269.

Vergauwen, R. (2014) Mysterianism Revisited: On the Semiotics of Consciousness, in Allo, P. and Van Kerkhove, B. (Eds.), *Modestly radical or radically modest: Festschrift for Jean Paul Van Bendegem on the Occasion of his 60th Birthday,* pp. 179-209, College Publications.

Appendix: The Video and Presentation links:

Speaker	Presentation	Video
John Holland	http://www.paralimes.ntu.edu.sg/NewsnEvents/east-west/Documents/John%20Holland_slides.pdf	https://www.youtube.com/watch?v=lQvmLwj7zKE&index=10&list=PLasWJveXPWTEMVgZ1ieoc5whp4t7NKG_y&nohtml5=False
Jean-Pierre Changeux*	http://www.paralimes.ntu.edu.sg/NewsnEvents/east-west/Documents/Jean-Pierre%20CHANGEUX_slides.pdf	https://www.youtube.com/watch?v=68WcH1hWkas&index=2&list=PLasWJveXPWTEMVgZ1ieoc5whp4t7NKG_y
Stan Gielen	https://www.youtube.com/watch?v=Qo6PLplfWlQ&list=PLasWJveXPWTEG1wvaoNqf56kA-PZN8_kl&index=6	http://www.paralimes.ntu.edu.sg/NewsnEvents/WorkshopEastWestConnectionsCulturalPatterns%2cCognitivePatternsandaGoodLife/Documents/Stan%20Gielen.pdf
Szabolcs Keri	http://www.paralimes.ntu.edu.sg/NewsnEvents/east-west/Documents/Szabolcs%20Keri_slides.pdf	https://www.youtube.com/watch?v=WQY8OkG2j1c&list=PLasWJveXPWTEMVgZ1ieoc5whp4t7NKG_y&index=6
Csaba Pleh	https://www.youtube.com/watch?v=KNsNOuB56ll&index=4&list=PLasWJveXPWTEG1wvaoNqf56kA-PZN8_kl	http://www.paralimes.ntu.edu.sg/NewsnEvents/WorkshopEastWestConnectionsCulturalPatterns%2cCognitivePatternsandaGoodLife/Documents/Csaba%20Pl%c3%a9h%20_%20Ottilia%20Boross.pdf